THE SOBER TRUTH

ALSO BY LANCE DODES

Breaking Addiction: A 7-Step Handbook for Ending Any Addiction

The Heart of Addiction: A New Approach to Understanding and Managing Alcoholism and Other Addictive Behaviors

THE SOBER TRUTH

DEBUNKING THE BAD SCIENCE BEHIND
12-STEP PROGRAMS AND THE REHAB INDUSTRY

LANCE DODES, MD
AND ZACHARY DODES

Beacon Press
Boston

BEACON PRESS
Boston, Massachusetts
www.beacon.org

Beacon Press books
are published under the auspices of
the Unitarian Universalist Association of Congregations.

Many names and identifying characteristics of the patients
mentioned in this work have been changed to protect their identities.

17 16 15 14   8 7 6 5 4 3 2 1

This book is printed on acid-free paper that meets the uncoated paper
ANSI/NISO specifications for permanence as revised in 1992.

Text design and composition by Kim Arney

Library of Congress Cataloging-in-Publication Data
Dodes, Lance M.
The sober truth : debunking the bad science behind 12-step programs
and the rehab industry / Lance Dodes, MD and Zachary Dodes.
        pages   cm
Includes bibliographical references.
ISBN 978-0-8070-3315-9 (hardcover : alk. paper)
ISBN 978-0-8070-3316-6 (ebook)
1. Twelve-step programs. 2. Addicts—Rehabilitation.
3. Substance abuse—Treatment. I. Dodes, Zachary, 1976– II. Title.
HV4998.D634 2014
616.86'06—dc23
2013043331

For the many people who struggle daily with addiction, their families, and friends, and for our wonderful wives, Connie and Farrah.

CONTENTS

PREFACE

ALCOHOLICS ANONYMOUS WAS PROCLAIMED the correct treatment for alcoholism over seventy-five years ago despite the absence of any scientific evidence of the approach's efficacy, and we have been on the wrong path ever since. Today, almost every treatment center, physician, and court system in the country uses this model. Yet it has one of the worst success rates in all of medicine: between 5 and 10 percent, hardly better than no treatment at all.

Most of the expensive, famous rehab centers that base their treatment on the Twelve Steps likewise have offered no evidence for their effectiveness. Most of them don't even study their own outcomes.

One would hope we could turn to science for careful studies of AA and its effectiveness. But science has failed us: the AA question was considered settled almost before it was asked, and what studies exist that claim to substantiate AA have been riddled with problems in both methodology and analysis. Nobody has ever carefully and rigorously reviewed these studies and reported the results to the public. In this book, we do just that.

The failure of addiction treatment in our country is especially discouraging since there are better ways to both understand addiction and treat it, and it's costing us thousands of lives and billions of dollars. With this book, we hope to begin a more productive conversation.

A Note About Format This book was written by both of us, but because Lance has devoted his career to understanding addiction, we have decided to write it in the first person. Zachary's equal contributions are everywhere, however, from the quality of the writing to his sharp understanding of good and bad science. Neither of us could have written this book alone.

CHAPTER ONE

THE PROBLEM

ALCOHOLICS ANONYMOUS IS A part of our nation's fabric. In the seventy-six years since AA was created, 12-step programs have expanded to include over three hundred different organizations, focusing on such diverse issues as smoking, shoplifting, social phobia, debt, recovery from incest, even vulgarity. All told, more than five million people recite the Serenity Prayer at meetings across the United States every year.

Twelve-step programs hold a privileged place in our culture as well. The legions of "anonymous" members who comprise these groups are helped in their proselytizing mission by hit TV shows such as *Intervention*, which preaches the gospel of recovery. "Going to rehab" is likewise a common refrain in music and film, where it is almost always uncritically presented as the one true hope for beating addiction. AA and rehab have even been codified into our legal system: court-mandated attendance, which began in the late 1980s, is today a staple of drug-crime policy. Every year, our state and federal governments spend over $15 billion on substance-abuse treatment for addicts, the vast majority of which are based on 12-step programs.[1] There is only one problem: these programs almost always fail.

Peer-reviewed studies peg the success rate of AA somewhere between 5 and 10 percent. That is, about one of every fifteen people who enter these programs is able to become and stay sober. In 2006, one of the most prestigious scientific research organizations in the world, the Cochrane Collaboration, conducted a review of the many studies conducted between 1966 and 2005 and reached a stunning conclusion: "No experimental studies unequivocally demonstrated the effectiveness of AA" in treating alcoholism.[2] This group reached the same conclusion about professional AA-oriented treatment (12-step facilitation therapy, or TSF), which is the core of virtually every alcoholism-rehabilitation program in the country.

Many people greet this finding with open hostility. After all, walk down any street in any city and you are likely to run into a dozen people who swear by AA—either from personal experience or because they know someone whose life was saved by the program. Even people who have no experience with AA may still have heard that it works or protest that 5 to 10 percent is a significant number when we're talking about millions of people. *So AA isn't perfect*, runs this thread of reasoning. *Have you got anything better?*

There are good answers to these objections, and they will take up a considerable portion of this book. For now, I will simply say that there are indeed better treatments for addiction—but the issues with AA's approach run far deeper than its statistical success rate. While it's praiseworthy that some do well in AA, the problem is that our society has followed AA's lead in presuming that 12-step treatment is good for the other 90 percent of people with addictions.

Any substantive conversation about treatment in this country must reckon with the toll levied when a culture encourages one approach to the exclusion of all others, especially when that culture limits the treatment options for suffering people, ignores advances in understanding addiction, and excludes and even shames the great majority of people who fail in the sanctioned approach.

THE AA MONOPOLY

AA began as a nonprofessional attempt to grapple with the alcoholism of its founders. It arose and took its famous twelve steps directly from the Oxford Group, a fundamentalist religious organization founded in the early twentieth century. It came to life on the day that its founder, Bill Wilson, witnessed a "bright flash of light" in a hospital room.

Although the fledgling organization lacked any scientific backing, research, or clinical experience to support its method, AA spread like wildfire through a country desperate for hope at the end of Prohibition and in the midst of the Great Depression. It soon became immaterial whether AA worked well or worked at all: it had claimed its place as the last best hope for beating the mighty specter of addiction. It had become the indispensable treatment, the sine qua non of addiction recovery in the United States. And science looked away.

AA has managed to survive, in part, because members who become and remain sober speak and write about it regularly. This is no accident: AA's twelfth step expressly tells members to proselytize for the organization: "Having had a spiritual awakening as the result of these Steps, we tried to carry this message to alcoholics, and to practice these principles in all our affairs." Adherence to this step has created a classic sampling error: because most of us hear only from the people who succeeded in the program, it is natural to conclude that they represent the whole. In reality, these members speak for an exceptionally small percentage of addicts, as we will see.

Beyond these individual proselytizing efforts, AA makes inflated claims about itself. Its foundational document, *Alcoholics Anonymous* (commonly referred to as the "Big Book" and a perennial best seller), spells out a confident ethos regularly endorsed by AA members:

> Rarely have we seen a person fail who has thoroughly followed our path. Those who do not recover are people who cannot or will not completely give themselves to this simple program, usually men and women who are constitutionally incapable of being honest with themselves. There are such unfortunates. They are not at fault; they seem to have been born that way. They are naturally incapable of grasping and developing a manner of living which demands rigorous honesty. Their chances are less than average. There are those, too, who suffer from grave emotional and mental disorders, but many of them do recover if they have the capacity to be honest.[3]

In other words, the program doesn't fail; *you* fail.

Imagine if similar claims were made in defense of an ineffective antibiotic. Imagine dismissing millions of people who did not respond to a new form of chemotherapy as "constitutionally incapable" of properly receiving the drug. Of course, no researchers would make such claims in scientific circles—if they did, they would risk losing their standing. In professional medicine, if a treatment doesn't work, it's the treatment that must be scrutinized, not the patient. Not so for Alcoholics Anonymous.

WALKING THE TWELVE STEPS

More than anything, AA offers a comforting veneer of actionable change: it is something you can *do*. Twelve steps sounds like science; it feels like rigor; it has the syntax of a roadmap. Yet when we examine these twelve steps more closely, we find dubious ideas and even some potentially harmful myths.

Step 1: "We admitted we were powerless over alcohol, that our lives had become unmanageable."

This step sounds appealing to some and grates heavily on others. The notion of declaring powerlessness is intended to evoke a sense of surrender that might give way to spiritual rebirth. Compelling as this is as a narrative device, it lacks any clinical merit or scientific backing. I'll examine this more closely in the chapters ahead.

Step 2: "Came to believe that a Power greater than ourselves could restore us to sanity."

Many scholars have written about the close bond between AA and religion. This is perhaps inevitable: AA was founded as a religious organization whose design and practices hewed closely to its spiritual forerunner, the Oxford Group, whose members believed strongly in the purging of sinfulness through conversion experiences. As Bill Wilson wrote in the Big Book: "To some people we need not, and probably should not, emphasize the spiritual feature on our first approach. We might prejudice them. At the moment we are trying to put our lives in order. But this is not an end in itself. Our real purpose is to fit ourselves to be of maximum service to God."[4]

Religion can have a salutary effect on people in crisis, of course, and its strong emphasis on community bonds is often indispensable. But do these comforting feelings address the causes of addiction or lead to permanent recovery in any meaningful way? As we will see, the evidence is scant.

Step 3: "Made a decision to turn our will and our lives over to the care of God as we understood God."

For an organization that has expressly denied religious standing and publicly claims a secular—even scientific—approach, it is curious that AA retains these explicit references to a spiritual power whose care might help light the way toward recovery. Even for addicts who opt to interpret this step secularly, the problem persists: why can't this ultimate power lie within the addict?

Step 4: "Made a searching and fearless moral inventory of ourselves."

The notion that people with addictions suffer from a failure of morality to be indexed and removed is fundamental to Alcoholics Anonymous. Yet addiction is not a moral defect, and to suggest that does a great disservice to people suffering with this disorder.

Step 5: "Admitted to God, to ourselves, and to another human being the exact nature of our wrongs."

Step 6: "Were entirely ready to have God remove all these defects of character."

Step 7: "Humbly asked God to remove our shortcomings."

These steps rehash the problems of their predecessors: the religiosity, the admission of moral defectiveness, the embrace of powerlessness, and the search for a cure through divine purification. The degradation woven through these steps also seems unwittingly designed to exacerbate, rather than relieve, the humiliating feelings so common in addiction. If moral self-flagellation could cure addiction, we could be sure there would be precious few addicts.

Step 8: "Made a list of all persons we had harmed and became willing to make amends to them all."

Step 9: "Made direct amends to such people wherever possible, except when to do so would injure them or others."

There is nothing inherently wrong with apologizing to those who have been harmed, directly or indirectly, by the consequences of addiction. The problem is the echo once more of the fundamentalist religious principle: that the path to recovery is to cleanse oneself of sin. Yes, apologies can be powerful things, and there's no question that reconciling with people can be a liberating and uplifting experience. But grounding this advice within a framework of treatment alters its timbre, transforming an elective act into one of penance.

Step 10: "Continued to take personal inventory, and when we were wrong promptly admitted it."

People suffering with addictions as a rule tend to be well aware of the many "wrongs" they have committed. Awareness of this fact doesn't help the problem.

Step 11: "Sought through prayer and meditation to improve our conscious contact with God as we understood God, praying only for knowledge of God's will for us and the power to carry that out."

If AA were simply presented as a religious movement dedicated to trying to comfort addicts through faith and prayer, the program would not be so problematic. What is troubling is how resolutely—and some might say disingenuously—AA has taken pains to dissociate itself from the faith-based methodology it encourages.

Step 12: "Having had a spiritual awakening as the result of these steps, we tried to carry this message to other addicts and to practice these principles in all our affairs."

AA's emphasis on proselytizing, a basic tool through which recognized religions and certain fringe religious groups spread their message, is an essential part of its worldwide success, and it's a big reason that it has been nearly impossible to have an open national dialogue about other, potentially better ways to treat addiction.

THE CONSEQUENCES OF BAD TREATMENT

I have been treating people suffering with addictions in public and private hospitals, in clinics, and in my private practice for more than thirty years. In that time, I have met and listened to a very large number of people who have "failed" at AA and some who continue to swear by it, despite repeated recidivism.

Dominic's case is just one example (I have changed the names and nonessential details in the passage below and whenever I discuss patients in this book). Dominic began drinking heavily as a junior at a good college. Weekly binges soon turned to daily abuse, with predictable results: his grades plummeted; his attendance vanished. By the time he arrived home for winter break, Dominic's family was deeply concerned about his deterioration. They advised him to seek counseling at the university health center.

Advisors there recommended that Dominic begin attending AA, which he did. He became fond of his sponsor and felt included for the first time in years—no small feat for a suffering young man. But he also found himself increasingly resentful of the "tally system" that AA uses to measure sobriety: every time he "slipped" and had a drink, he "went back to zero." All the chips he'd earned—the tokens given by AA for milestone periods of sobriety—became meaningless. This system compounded his sense of shame and anger, leading him to wonder why he lacked the willpower or fortitude to master the incredible force of his alcoholism.

By spring, Dominic had dropped out of college. His parents turned to the family doctor for advice. She told him to double down on AA—to attend ninety meetings in ninety days, which is a common AA prescription.

It worked. Although many of the faces at the meetings kept changing and Dominic constantly felt the urge to drink, he found a few "old-timers" who believed wholly in the program and who encouraged him to dismiss the great majority of people who fell through the cracks. They just weren't ready to stop, he was reassured. Dominic soon learned to distract himself from thinking about alcohol and to call his sponsor when the urge arose.

Four months into the program, Dominic became frustrated dur-ing a call with his bank. He bought a fifth of vodka and drank so much that he fell down the stairs, suffering three cracked vertebrae. A series of increasingly expensive stints in rehab followed throughout his twenties, with poor results. During this time, he was hospitalized twice and lost every job he held. A brief marriage ended in a bad divorce, and Dominic was deeply depressed by the time someone in his life recommended that he try something other than a 12-step program. Maybe talk therapy was worth a try.

When Dominic entered my office, he had accepted as empirical truth that he was a deeply flawed individual: amoral, narcissistic, and unable to turn himself over to a Higher Power. How else to explain the swath of destruction he had cut through his own life and the lives of those who loved him? His time in AA had also taught him that his deeper psychological life was immaterial to mastering his addiction. He had a disease; the solution was in the Twelve Steps. When he was ready to quit, he would.

It took eight months of psychotherapy before Dominic stopped drinking for good. Although he remained in therapy for several years after that, the key that unlocked his addiction was nothing more com-plex or ethereal than an understanding of what his addiction really was and how it really worked.

Dominic had felt enormously pressured all of his life, consumed by a suffocating need to excel in every activity. He was driven by a hunger to be "good enough"—accomplished enough, successful enough—to please his demanding father and blameful mother. Whenever he felt he was not performing up to his potential, his old sense of being trapped by implacable demands arose, and with it came a deep sense of shame and an equal fury at the awful helplessness he felt about this burden. Those were the moments he had to have a drink.

Eventually he came to realize that this odd coping mechanism made a certain kind of sense. By making a decision to drink, he was empowering himself—he no longer felt helpless. Once he understood the connection between his lifelong feelings and his urges to drink, he was able to view them with some perspective for the first time. He found that he was able to predict when his drive to drink would return, since it always tended to surface right after that old, unbearable pressure to perform. He developed enough awareness into what was beneath these urges that he could take a step back and deal with those issues more directly and appropriately. Over time, he was also able to work out the underlying narrative forces that had led him to feel so helpless throughout his life. He had, in other words, supplanted the notion of a Higher Power with something far more personally empowering: sophisticated self-awareness.

THE REHAB FICTION

Dominic's history follows the same contours as thousands of others. But one part of his story warrants special attention: the series of failed attempts at rehabilitation. Dominic's family lost close to $200,000— their total retirement savings—on this string of ineffectual programs.

Rehab owns a special place in the American imagination. Our nation invented the "Cadillac" rehab, manifested in such widely celebrated brand names as Hazelden, Sierra Tucson, and the Betty Ford Center. Ask the average American about any of these institutions and you will likely hear a response tinged with reverence—these are the standard-bearers, our front line against addiction. The fact that they are all extraordinarily expensive is almost beside the point: these rehabs are fighting the good fight, and they deserve every penny we've got.

Unfortunately, nearly all these programs use an adaptation of the same AA approach that has been shown repeatedly to be highly ineffective. Where they deviate from traditional AA dogma is actually more alarming: many top rehab programs include extra features such as horseback riding, Reiki massage, and "adventure therapy" to help their clients exorcise the demons of addiction. Some renowned programs even have "equine therapists" available to treat addiction—a fairly novel credential in this context, to put it kindly. Sadly, there is no evidence that these additional "treatments" serve any purpose other than to provide momentary comfort to their clientele—and cover for the programs' astronomical fees, which can exceed $90,000 a month.

Why do we tolerate this industry? One reason may sound familiar: in rehab, one feels that one is *doing* something, taking on a life-changing intervention whose exorbitant expense ironically reinforces the impression that epochal changes must be just around the corner. It is marketed as the sort of cleansing experience that can herald the dawn of a new era. How many of us have not indulged this fantasy at one time or another—the daydream that if we could just put our lives "on pause" for a while and retreat somewhere pastoral and lovely, we could finally make sense of all our problems?

Alas, the effect is temporary at best. Many patients begin using again soon after they emerge from rehab, often suffering repeated relapses. The discouragement that follows these failures can magnify the desperation that originally brought them to help's door.

What's especially shocking is how the rehab industry responds to these individuals: they simply repeat their failed treatments, sometimes dozens of times. Repeat stays in rehab are very common, and readmission is almost always granted without any special consideration or review. On second and subsequent stays, the same program is offered, including lectures previously attended.

Any serious treatment center would study its own outcomes to modify and improve its approach. But rehabs generally don't do this. For example, only one of the three best-known facilities has ever published outcome studies (Hazelden); neither Betty Ford nor Sierra Tucson has checked to see if their treatment is producing any results for at least the past decade. Hazelden's follow-up studies looked at just the first year following discharge and showed disappointing results, as we will see later.

Efforts by journalists to solicit data from rehabs have also been met with resistance, making an independent audit of their results almost impossible and leading to the inevitable conclusion that the rest of the programs either don't study their own outcomes or refuse to publish what they find.[5]

CHAPTER TWO

THE RISE OF AA

AA IS UNDENIABLY AN international phenomenon, but its rise to world consciousness was neither easy nor inevitable. The story of AA's ascendance and ability to beat out so many competing ideas is a tale of tremendous will and effort that rests largely on the shoulders of its tireless messengers—none more so than AA founder Bill Wilson, known in recovery circles simply as "Bill W."

Bill Wilson was a lifelong alcoholic with a string of business failures under his belt before he managed to marshal America's most august institutions to the cause of AA. These included such household names as the Rockefeller family, the *Saturday Evening Post*, Yale University, and later, the American Medical Association. Some of this lobbying occurred in the open, in the form of public testimony and press, but a greater portion took the form of private navigation among the power players of America's medical elite.

To tell the story of AA's ascendancy properly, we must begin at the beginning and ask a simple question: What did people *do* about alcoholism before the advent of AA?

BEFORE AA: DARKNESS AND DIPSOMANIA

Alcoholism has almost certainly been with us for as long as alcohol itself. Fermented fruits, primitive spirits, and home-brewed wine feature broadly in indigenous rituals, and some of the earliest writings in Eastern and Western literature make reference to prodigious drinking.

A landmark essay in 1774, "Mighty Destroyer Destroyed," discussed alcoholism for the first time in American letters.[1] This was followed a decade later by Dr. Benjamin Rush's "Inquiry into the Effects of Ardent

Spirits on the Human Mind and Body," a widely circulated monograph that sought to describe "chronic drunkenness" from a scientific perspective, and to redefine the problem as a disease worth treating. This second essay became something of a foundational document for one of the more powerful political moments in American culture: the temperance movement.[2]

The term *temperance* was shorthand for a religiously inflected approach to the problem of "chronic drunkenness," one that held that alcohol itself was dangerous and addictive. More focused on drinking than on drinkers, the temperance movement gained momentum as a mass effort to rid homes and taverns of alcohol and, expressly, to restore morality to America. Protestants and Catholics alike endorsed different versions of the platform, and more than a million people had signed on with the movement by 1837.

None of these advocates seems to have spent much time seeking to lighten the burden of the "incurable drunk." The era's prevailing treatments consisted of detoxification, hospitalization, institutionalization, and prayer. But Americans wouldn't have long to wait for an innovation that might serve the "drunks" themselves; a major breakthrough was just around the corner.

In 1879, an Irish émigré named Dr. Leslie Keeley made a startling announcement: "Drunkenness is a disease, and I can cure it." The statement electrified the nation. Keeley had a secret sauce, a "tonic" of chemicals administered via injection, which he claimed had the ability to eradicate the craving for alcohol. Not much is known about these injections today, but some historians have speculated that they contained a mixture of "atropine, strychnine, cinchona [basically quinine], glycerin, and gold and sodium chloride." This was a tonic that, as one modern historian noted, required one "to possess a strong constitution to withstand the treatment."[3] Keeley was nonetheless famously bullish on his eponymous cure, telling anyone who would listen that it had no injurious effects, and that it worked 95 percent of the time.[4]

The Keeley method spawned a cottage industry of Keeley Institutes—some 120 nationwide—that would eventually "treat" as many as 500,000 alcoholics between 1880 and 1920. Alas, despite the storied fortitude required to withstand Keeley's needle, alcoholism itself was more than up to the task. Keeley's method fell out of favor as the public eventually recognized it as a scam. His branded network of rehab centers was completely shut down by the end of World War I.

Contemporaneous with Keeley's clinics was a rise in so-called *inebriate hospitals*—institutions dedicated specifically to drying out alcoholics. These institutions' philosophy, not so different from today's rehabilitation facilities, was that people could detoxify, heal, and eventually flourish if they were deprived of any alcohol for a period of time, often up to one year. But the inebriate hospitals were somewhat different from today's palatial rehabs in one important way: patients were often subjected to cold showers and typically housed alongside society's cast-offs—the blind, those suffering from syphilis, the mentally ill, orphans, even prisoners.[5]

The inebriate hospitals also adopted another new procedure for alcoholism: prefrontal lobotomy. This, painfully, failed to cure the "disease" of alcoholism, with one account famously relating that, "[f]ollowing the procedure, the patient dressed and, pulling a hat down over his bandaged head, slipped out of the hospital in search of a drink."[6]

The nation soon lost its appetite for these pernicious facilities, and most of them closed by the end of the nineteenth century. Many alcoholics were consequently forced to seek help wherever they could, often in the "foul wards" of public hospitals as well as insane asylums.

Just as private institutions devoted to specific alcoholism treatment began to disappear, American legislation was seeking new ways to vilify drinking as a moral weakness and societal scourge. Various state laws passed between 1907 and 1913 called for "the mandatory sterilization of 'defectives': the mentally ill, the developmentally disabled, and alcoholics and addicts."[7] Then in 1919, a watershed: the Eighteenth Amendment was passed, enshrining into law a nationwide prohibition on the sale of alcohol. Any promising treatments that may have arisen between that day and the amendment's repeal in 1931 were almost certainly doomed to obscurity, as nobody could legally be said to be purchasing and drinking alcohol on a regular basis. Overnight, a public health issue became a legal one, and the public's appetite for treatment seems to have collapsed. Even the popular *Journal of Inebriety* shuttered during this era, erasing one of the only scholarly forums on the causes and treatment of alcohol addiction.[8]

At the threshold of AA's invention, America carried a population of alcoholics deeply fatigued by many decades of barbaric treatment, imprisonment, and isolation; rattled by errant snake oil "cures"; and suffused with a widespread sense of hopelessness. Bill Wilson was just such an alcoholic.

BILL'S STORY

Although Bill Wilson would later become the primary architect of Alcoholics Anonymous, it was many years before he came to acknowledge his drinking addiction, and even longer before the famous religious conversion experience that led to the creation of AA. Given his essential role, it is useful to consider the man himself—not just for what his life has to teach us about AA, but for its power as an example of one man's descent into the agony of alcoholism.

William Griffith Wilson was born on November 26, 1895. He came from a moderately well-to-do Vermont family, raised in a home large and impressive enough that it would later become a country inn. But Wilson's home life was chaotic, and his childhood was scarred by a series of wrenching abandonments.

Nearly every man in Wilson's family had a drinking problem. Wilson's grandfather, widely known for his alcohol consumption, struggled with addiction for most of his life, signing popular promises of the day known as "Temperance Pledges" on more than one occasion. Like many men of his time, he was also bamboozled by a series of traveling revival-tent preachers who arrived promising absolution and salvation from drinking via the power of the Lord.

Nothing worked until the fateful day when Wilson's grandfather had, by his telling, a miraculous conversion experience: "[I]n a desperate state one morning, he climbed to the top of Mount Aeolus. There, after beseeching God to help him, he saw a blinding light and felt the wind of the Spirit. It was an experience that left him feeling so transformed that he practically ran down the mountain and into town."[9]

the house reported seeing him struggling to decide whether he should take oxygen or smoke another cigarette. The cigarette won every time.

A similar pattern arose around a different behavior: serial adultery. Wilson's need to sleep with women outside his marriage was legendary—so much so that AA members eventually put together a "Founder's Watch" committee designed to steer him away from any tempting young women at the numerous events he attended." Tellingly, one of Wilson's close friends noted the utter helplessness Wilson evinced in the face of what appears clearly to have been a sexual compulsion: "I think that was the worst part of it," [the friend] said. "Bill would always agree with me. "'I know,' he'd say. 'You're right.' Then, just when I would think we were finally getting somewhere, he would say, 'But I can't give it up.'" These multiple compulsive behaviors, including alcoholism, smoking, and sexuality, foreshadow our later understanding of addiction as being a global problem not restricted to any particular substance or behavior.

Throughout his life, Wilson also suffered with bouts of depression. These episodes were frequent and paralyzing and would hound him until his death with overwhelming feelings of worthlessness and hopelessness. Once alcohol was no longer in the picture, Wilson turned to faith as a salve for these feelings. He would find temporary relief under the care of Father Edward Dowling, who "compared Bill's malaise to that of the saints." (Dowling would later go on to write the first Catholic endorsement of AA; he was especially impressed by the Big Book's parallels to the Spiritual Exercises of St. Ignatius Loyola.) Wilson never wavered from his conviction that his depression was caused by "a lack of faith."

The question of Wilson's faith has suffused AA's history, and has regularly come up as a point of concern and confusion. Some insight may be gleaned from Wilson's own writings.

Wilson may have experienced ambivalence about the ideal form and structure of his belief system, but unalloyed faith was fundamental to him. Wilson claimed that "God was the source of the goodness and guidance alcoholics could rely on to help them put an end to their drinking and restore wholeness to their lives." He maintained that people

Wilson's grandfather's "miracle" became the stuff of legend in
He never drank again.

Bill Wilson grew up heavily influenced by his grandfather, espec
so because his parents divorced and his father moved away when
son was just eleven. It would be nine years before Wilson saw his fa
again. During this period, his mother left him as well, never return
for longer than a short visit.

Wilson had his own way of managing the feelings associated w
his parents' dual abandonment. Many accounts of his formative yea
describe a fierce defensiveness against his peers and an overweenir
desire to "prove himself"—by force if necessary—whether or not an
judgment had been directed his way. If Wilson could be described a
an angry person, however, there is one direction in which he seemed
never to direct his resentment: "Astonishingly, Wilson never blamed his
father for his absence or expressed any anger toward him" for abandon-
ing his family for nine years, without correspondence or child support
of any kind.

Wilson's pain showed itself in other ways. He struggled in school and
swung between significant highs and lows in morale. Securing a popular
girlfriend in high school began an upward cycle of contentment that
saw him named class president, but her death during emergency sur-
gery devastated him, sending him into a deep depression. Wilson also
suffered from occasional panic attacks, which left him convinced that
he had a heart condition. As a consequence, he failed nearly every physical test he was given after eventually matriculating to military college.
He suffered through many years of listlessness and deep melancholy.

Wilson also struggled with controlling his behavior. As his biographer put it, "Bill was compulsive, given to emotional extremes. . . . Even
after he stopped drinking, he was still a heavy consumer of cigarettes
and coffee. He had a sweet tooth, a large appetite for sex, and a major
enthusiasm for LSD and, later, for niacin, a B-complex vitamin."

Indeed, he was such a heavy smoker that the effects of tobacco would
rob him of his mobility and, eventually, his life. One account recalls that
he continued to smoke even in his old age when he needed frequent
doses of oxygen just to make it through the day. Friends who arrived at

who doubted the existence of God "were standing with their backs to the light." He never doubted the presence of a miraculous divine spirit in his own famous conversion experience, which closely mimicked his grandfather's: Wilson "felt lifted up, as though the great clean wind of a mountain top blew through and through."

Yet if Wilson's embrace of religion was absolute, it was also eclectic and fungible. He once famously described himself as "a shopper at the theological pie counter." He dabbled in Christian Science at one point and Catholicism at another. He and his wife, Lois, hosted a number of séances, which they called "spooking sessions," throughout the 1940s and '50s; Lois would later claim with pride that they levitated the table "on a number of occasions." She also liked to tell about Wilson's spiritual powers, bragging about gifts such as automatic writing, something that reportedly meant a great deal to him.

It is essentially impossible to separate Wilson's passion for the spiritual from his founding of AA, despite the organization's frequent protestations that it is nonreligious in nature. Of course, Alcoholics Anonymous members have every possible view about religion. But the organization is clearly permeated with Wilson's religious beliefs.

Wilson himself said twenty years following his conversion that he "wanted every alcoholic to be able to say, as he could, that their belief in God was 'no longer a question of faith' but 'the certainty of knowledge [gained] through evidence.'"

THE ROOTS OF AA

The teenaged Bill Wilson was feeling characteristically unhappy when he had his first drink at a reception for Officer Candidate School in Bedford, Massachusetts. The effect, his biographer recounts, was instantaneous: "[A]lcohol produced in him instant feelings of completeness, invulnerability, and an ecstasy that approached the religious." So began Wilson's long experience with drinking.

Wilson's early struggles with alcohol led him to numerous humiliations. He lost several jobs and most of his friends, and checked into a local hospital several times in hopes of shaking his affliction. In 1934, Wilson was approached about joining the Oxford Group, a religious organization bent on creating a moral realignment in America by facilitating spiritual rebirth through miraculous conversion experiences. Wilson's friend Ebby Thacher, who brought him into the fold, had achieved sobriety through the organization and thought Wilson might do the same.

Wilson debated the merits of joining the Oxford Group over a period of months. His concerns were telling: "To keep drinking meant a certain alcoholic death or institutionalization, but stopping drinking by embracing religion seemed to be trading one odious dependency for another." Thacher pressed the case, recounting the tale of their mutual friend "Rowland P.," who had gone to Switzerland to seek care from Carl Jung. The eminent psychoanalyst had assured the man that his only hope lay in religion (Jung was a proponent of the mystical power of conversion experiences). Ebby Thacher also enjoined Wilson to read William James's *Varieties of Religious Experience*, a work that also endorsed spiritual conversion, stating "the only cure for dipsomania [alcoholism] is religiomania."[10]

When Wilson finally attended his first Oxford Group meeting, he approached the altar and pledged his life to Christ. He was back drinking the very next day. Yet a singular moment shortly thereafter would forever change his mind—and alter the history of alcohol treatment in the twentieth century. One day while lying prone and feeling despair during his fourth admission to Towns Hospital, Wilson is reported to have cried out, "I'll do anything! Anything at all! If there be a God, let Him show Himself!" He described seeing a bright light, feeling euphoric, then a great calm. Armed with the certitude and wonder that this moment produced in him, Wilson never drank again. It was a stark pivot point in his life.[11]

Wilson's story was a compelling one, but it wasn't terribly unusual for the era. Stories of conversion experiences were beacons of hope as the nation twisted in the horrors of the Great Depression. Americans had developed a newfound suspicion of the science that had delivered mechanization and its attendant layoffs, and an invigorated interest in the sublime. Yet Wilson's vision may have also been informed by more terrestrial factors. He rarely mentioned in retelling this story that he was being treated at the time by the "Belladonna Cure," a chemical cocktail that included the known hallucinogens atropine and scopolamine.

Perhaps more importantly, we should notice this story's startling similarity to his grandfather's. Just like the older man, Wilson claimed that he'd been transported to a mountaintop, where he experienced a nearly word-for-word reenactment of the same sensations—"uplift" and "spirit"—that his grandfather spoke about more or less continuously during Wilson's childhood.

Despite these clues that more prosaic forces may have been at work, Wilson believed for the rest of his life that he had been touched by God, and he was absolutely certain that divine experience had forever liberated him from the urge to drink.

Wilson rejoined the Oxford Group with evangelical zeal. He soon began to wonder if the organization's spiritual practices might be adapted as a universal cure for alcoholism. Looking back on this time, Wilson wrote: "The early AA got its ideas of self-examination, acknowledgment of character defects, restitution for harm done, and working with others straight from the Oxford Group and directly from Sam Shoemaker, their former leader in America, and from nowhere else."[12]

Although Wilson felt indebted to the Oxford Group for many things, he would eventually break from the organization. He was frequently dismayed by the group's lack of interest in alcoholics, as well as its increasing reliance on fame-seeking stunts. He also bristled at its repeated admonishments of his smoking and at a hierarchical structure that designated certain members "maximum" after they had attained a state of purity and seniority that others lacked.

One bedrock tenet of the Oxford Group, however, would influence AA for years to come: an absolute opposition to medical or psychological explanations for human failings and thus a complete prohibition on professional treatment of any kind.

AA IS BORN

AA is said to have been born when Bill Wilson met Dr. Bob Smith, who would eventually become Wilson's first successful sobriety effort. Wilson had tried to help many alcoholics before "Dr. Bob," but discovered to his exasperation that the story of his own miraculous conversion did not have the effect he desired. When a business trip took him to Akron, Ohio, however, he successfully made the case for spiritual rebirth for the first time to the doctor, whose drinking had shredded his life and practice.

Wilson and Smith soon joined forces to share their sobriety with others. They strongly believed that helping other people get sober had a salutary effect that flowed both ways: it would cure the "target" and it would help to shore up their own recovery. During this early stage in the organization's history, the two men also developed some theories of their own, including the notion that alcoholics were "in a state of insanity rather than a state of sin."[13] They soon systematized their outreach efforts:

> They would first approach the man's wife, and later they would approach the individual directly by going to his home or by inviting him to the Smiths' home. The objective was to get the man to surrender, and the surrender involved a confession of powerlessness and a prayer that said the man believed in a higher power and could be restored to sanity. This process would sometimes take place in the kitchen, or at other times it was at the man's bed with Wilson kneeling on one side of the bed and Smith on the other side. This way the man would be led to admit his defeat.[14]

This approach met with tremendous resistance. In one early internal audit, Wilson and Smith calculated their success rate at just 5 percent. Even many of those who seemed willing to listen and try returned to drinking.

Still, after a couple of years the two men felt encouraged: "Among those they had tried to help, the failures were endless, and many of those who seemed sincerely willing to try their approach were struggling. When they were done counting, though, they realized that between Akron and New York there were now forty alcoholics staying sober, and half of them had not had a drink for more than a year. Their program was working."

Wilson decided it was time to write a book.

THE BIG BOOK

When Bill Wilson sat down to write *Alcoholics Anonymous*, he first prayed for guidance. The Twelve Steps themselves reportedly came to him in a single inspiration. (He identified the number twelve with the Twelve Apostles, and felt that this was a fitting number.) Besides enumerating the steps for the first time, the "Big Book," as it came to be known, included a number of "case studies" describing the lives of early members who recovered with the help of AA. (Throughout his life, Wilson quietly kept track of those members whose experiences had been considered solid enough for inclusion in the book: about half of them had not remained sober.)

Wilson and his early acolytes promoted the book every chance they could. So devoted were AA's early members to burnishing the reputation of their fledgling organization, in fact, that when one member, Morgan R., secured an interview on a widely popular radio show, members kept him locked in a hotel room "for several days under 24 hour watch" out of fear that he would drink before the show. When the interview went off successfully, another early backer, Hank P., mailed twenty thousand postcards to doctors, urging them to purchase *Alcoholics Anonymous*.[15]

Despite these efforts, AA would not become widely known until a few years later, when two national articles were published in rapid succession. The first appeared in *Liberty*, a very popular magazine run by Fulton Oursler, an early Oxford Group member who would also later serve as a trustee of the Alcoholic Foundation, AA's governing body. The article was a glowing account of Wilson's organization. The writer, Morris Markey, called AA's method an overwhelming success, despite a notable absence of any evidence that might attest to such success. Subtitled "A Cure That Borders on the Miraculous—and It Works!," the piece relied heavily on sources of Wilson's choosing, especially Dr. William Silkworth, the physician at Towns Hospital who had been so impressed by Wilson's conversion that he gave him free rein to circulate among the patients.

"Within the last four years," Markey wrote, "evidence has appeared which has startled hard-boiled medical men by proving that the compulsion neurosis can be entirely eliminated." Describing how the organization approached new members, Markey wrote, "One or another of the members keeps working on him from day to day. And presently the miracle."

Silkworth, a supporter of AA from its inception, was quoted as well, assembling a motley collection of speculation and anecdote into a theory of his own:

> We all know that the alcoholic has an urge to share his troubles. . . . But the psychoanalyst, being of human clay, is not often a big enough man for that job. The patient simply cannot generate enough confidence in him. But the patient can have enough confidence in God—once he has gone through the mystical experience of recognizing God. And upon that principle the Alcoholic Foundation rests. The medical profession, in general, accepts the principle as sound.

This may have been true of some in the medical profession, but a representative opinion it was not. Yet Wilson and AA would go on to score an even greater public relations coup in the months that followed, when America's most widely read magazine, the *Saturday Evening Post*, ran a feature on March 1, 1941, written by Jack Alexander and called simply "Alcoholics Anonymous." It was so effusive and unqualified in its praise that copies are still circulated by AA members.

Alexander's writing took the form of a skeptic's journey from doubt to belief, a narrative that practically hums with enchantment—not just with AA's methods, but with its approach to living generally. (Alexander would also go on to become a trustee of the Alcoholic Foundation.)

Among other points, Alexander echoed and amplified the same antiprofessional message as the *Liberty* article, underscoring what remains a widely held belief among many AA members: that only an alcoholic can help another alcoholic: "A bridge of confidence is thereby erected, spanning a gap, which has baffled the physician, the minister, the priest, or the hapless relatives. . . . Only an alcoholic can squat on another alcoholic's chest for hours with the proper combination of discipline and sympathy." Alexander also waxed poetic about the rosy existence of those saved by AA, highlighting a parade of success stories. One extended passage memorably described the benefits of joining AA's nationwide brotherhood of bonhomie:

> For the Brewsters, the Martins, the Watkinses, the Tracys, and the other reformed alcoholics, congenial company is now available wherever they happen to be. In the larger cities, A.A.s meet one another daily at lunch in favored restaurants. The Cleveland groups give big parties on New Year's and other holidays, at which gallons of coffee and soft drinks are consumed. Chicago holds open house on Friday, Saturday and Sunday—alternating, on the North, West, and South Sides—so that no lonesome A.A. need revert to liquor over the weekend for lack of companionship. Some play cribbage or bridge, the winner of each hand contributing to a kitty for paying of entertainment expenses. The others listen to the radio, dance, eat, or just talk. All alcoholics, drunk or sober, like to gab. They are among the most society-loving people in the world, which may help to explain why they got to be alcoholics in the first place.

Fabulous life aside, the article also offered some uncited statistics. Over two thousand souls had been "saved by AA" to date, claimed Alexander, and the organization's success rate was without equal:

> One-hundred-percent effectiveness with non-psychotic drinkers who sincerely want to quit is claimed by the workers of Alcoholics Anonymous. The program will not work, they add, with those who only "want to want to quit," or who want to quit because they are afraid of losing their families or their jobs. The effective desire, they state, must be based upon enlightened self-interest; the applicant must want to get away from liquor to head off incarceration or premature death.

Alexander also pointed out one Philadelphia chapter that claimed an 87 percent success rate, once again without any confirmation.

There is but one mention of an opposing viewpoint anywhere in the feature, and it is quickly eclipsed before the author even finds his way to the end of the next sentence: "However, many doctors remain skeptical.

Dr. Foster Kennedy, an eminent New York neurologist, probably had these in mind when he stated at a meeting a year ago: 'The aim of those concerned in this effort against alcoholism is high; their success has been considerable; and I believe medical men of goodwill should aid.'"

Alexander closed the piece with a description of Bill and Lois Wilson's life that bordered on hagiography: "In a manner reminiscent of the primitive Christians, they have moved about, finding shelter in the home of A.A. colleagues and sometimes wearing borrowed clothing."

The article was a sensation. It drew six thousand letters from around the world, all of which the *Post* promptly forwarded to the Alcoholism Foundation. By the end of that year, the *Ladies' Home Journal* had published a similarly glowing piece and AA had been featured in a gushing "March of Time" newsreel shown throughout the nation.[16]

ALCOHOLICS ANONYMOUS ENTERS THE ESTABLISHMENT

AA's members recognized early on that to establish true legitimacy, they would eventually need to earn the imprimatur of the scientific community. The process was hardly smooth. When the Big Book was first published in 1939, the American Medical Association, bewildered by its tone and inflated claims, called the work "a curious combination of organizing propaganda and religious exhortation. . . . [T]he one valid thing in the book is the recognition of the seriousness of addiction to alcohol. Other than this, the book has no scientific merit or interest."[17]

The *Journal of Nervous and Mental Diseases* went even further in 1940, calling AA a "regressive mass psychological method" and a "religious fervor," writing: "The big, big book, *i.e.* big in words, is a rambling sort of camp-meeting confession of experiences, told in the form of biographies of various alcoholics who had been to a certain institution and have provisionally recovered, chiefly under the influence of the 'big brothers of the spirit.' Of the inner meaning of alcoholism there is hardly a word. It is all surface material."

Undeterred, AA wouldn't have long to wait before one of its own had discovered a way to influence the establishment from within. Marty Mann, a wealthy Chicago debutante, was among the first women ever to join Alcoholics Anonymous. Her own conversion story describes being struck instantly and irrevocably by a passage in the Big Book, "We cannot live with anger"—a phrase that reportedly produced in her an immediate and life-altering sense of calm. Not content to simply spread the word one-to-one as the twelfth step recommends, Mann became an active force in lobbying for the group on a national stage. Her breakthrough came when she formed the National Council on Alcoholism and Drug Dependence, an advocacy group that is still active. Under the aegis of this newly formed organization, Mann testified many times in front of medical communities, often without disclosing her status as a member of Alcoholics Anonymous.

In 1943 Marty Mann and Bill Wilson had joined forces with another major figure—E. M. Jellinek—to establish a new institution at one of the nation's most prestigious schools: Yale University. Wilson himself was placed on the faculty.

Jellinek, an important figure in his own right, is considered the primary author of the "disease theory" of alcoholism, which holds that heavy drinking is in some substantive way different from other behaviors—that rather than being a behavior, it is in fact a gradually progressive disease analogous to other chronic medical illnesses. His model of inevitable deterioration was soon disproven (Jellinek ultimately distanced himself from it), but AA embraced it. Even today, AA members regularly repeat the mantra that continued drinking leads inevitably to insanity and death.

It was perhaps unexpected that AA would fasten onto Jellinek's view, given that the physician's model of alcoholism as a medical disease did not precisely comport with the organization's own model of alcoholism as a spiritual illness. But throughout AA's history, its members have often embraced any literature that references disease, whether degenerative, genetic, or biochemical. AA favors the term *disease* because it fits with the description of alcoholism as a disease in its own literature. It also supports the foundational notion that an addict's behavior is uncontrollable ("We admitted we were powerless over alcohol"). Ultimately the mechanism of the disease (and whether it is strictly logical to embrace it, given AA's own views) has been less important than the word itself.

Jellinek's landmark paper establishing his ideas was published in 1946.[18] It went on to be heavily cited in the years to come—despite the fact that it was based on a study funded by Marty Mann and another backer and employed just ninety-eight questionnaires returned by self-selected members of AA who had seen them in the *Grapevine*, AA's own magazine.[19]

AA'S SPREADING INFLUENCE

In 1951, largely on the strength of self-reported success and popular articles, AA was honored with the Lasker Award, "given by the American Public Health Association for outstanding achievement in the fields of medical research or public health administration." The citation makes no mention of any scientific study that might prove or disprove the organization's efficacy, simply declaring its "recognition of [AA's] unique and highly successful approach" to alcoholism.

AA's march toward public legitimacy accelerated. In 1955, at AA's annual conference in Missouri, Dr. W. W. Bauer, an eminent member of the American Medical Association, told the assembled crowd: "You who have seen what alcohol can do in your lives are working together in groups and individually, and you are making a bigger impression on the problem of alcohol than has ever been made before." Harry Tiebout, Wilson's personal therapist, also appeared, assuring the collected members that AA was "not just a miracle but a way of life which is filled with eternal value."[20]

It wasn't long before the court systems began to mandate AA attendance for drug and alcohol offenders. AA won a landmark decision in 1966 when two decisions from a federal appeals court upheld the disease concept of alcoholism and the court's use of it, despite the fact that there was scant precedent for a US court of law to assign itself the power of medical diagnosis. Although later decisions would rule court-mandated 12-step attendance unconstitutional, judges still refer people to AA as part of sentencing or as a condition of probation. Dr. Arthur Horvath, a past president of the Division on Addictions of the American Psychological Association, summarizes the current legal status of this practice:

If you have been convicted of an offense related to addiction, it is common to be ordered to attend support groups, treatment, or both. It has also been common that you would be ordered, not just to a support group, but to Alcoholics Anonymous (AA) specifically, or to another 12-step based group.

Based on recent court decisions, if you have been ordered to attend a 12-step group or 12-step based treatment by the government (the order could be coming from a court, prison officer, probation or parole officer, licensing board or licensing board diversion program, or anyone authorized to act on behalf of the government), you have the right *not* to attend them. However, you can still be required to attend some form of support group, and some type of treatment.

These court decisions are based on the finding that AA is religious enough that being required to attend it would be similar to requiring someone to attend church. Five US Circuit Courts of Appeal (the 2nd, 3rd, 7th, 8th, and 9th) have made similar rulings. . . . The 2nd Circuit Court decision states that AA "placed a heavy emphasis on spirituality and prayer, in both conception and in practice," that participants were told to "pray to God," and that meetings began and adjourned with "group prayer." The court therefore had "no doubt" that AA meetings were "intensely religious events." Although some have suggested that AA is spiritual but not religious, the court found AA to be religious.[21]

In 1966, President Lyndon Johnson proclaimed to the nation that "[t]he alcoholic suffers from a disease which will yield eventually to scientific research and adequate treatment."[22] The disease theory and AA's lobbying had at this point become difficult to separate. In 1970, Congress joined the consensus and passed a law known as the "Comprehensive Alcohol Abuse and Alcoholism Prevention Treatment and Rehabilitation Act," which established the National Institute on Alcohol Abuse and Alcoholism (NIAAA). Among those testifying to the lawmakers in support of the bill were Marty Mann and Bill Wilson.

In 1973, the "millionth copy" of *Alcoholics Anonymous* was presented to President Richard Nixon in the Oval Office. (AA is the only source for this number; to my knowledge, sales have never been publicly audited.)

According to the Federation of State Physician Health Programs, "By 1980 . . . all but three of the 54 U.S. medical societies of all states and jurisdictions had authorized or implemented impaired physician programs."[23] A recent paper looking at state-sponsored physician health groups (for doctors who have problems with addiction) found that "[r]egardless of setting or duration, essentially all treatment provided to these physicians (95%) was 12-step oriented."[24]

In 1989, the nation's first drug court appeared in Dade County, Florida. Its treatment plan was to remit nonviolent drug offenders to a 12-step program and to compel those who had failed follow-up drug tests to attend "supplementary" 12-step sessions.[25]

Examining this history, it is clear that AA has been extraordinarily effective at influencing public opinion and policy toward a favorable view of its ideas. What is missing from this account is notable as well: these strides were achieved without any triggering event, such as a well-designed study, that might support the organization's claims of efficacy. Most of AA's claims were simply grandfathered in, collecting legitimacy in a sort of echo chamber of reciprocal mentions that often featured the same handful of names.

CHAPTER THREE

DOES AA WORK?

WE COME NOW TO the essential question: *Is AA an effective treatment for alcoholism?* Many people have argued passionately on one side or the other of this debate, but these arguments are too often heated and anecdotal in nature. To truly determine whether and how often AA succeeds, we must examine the totality of the evidence and determine which studies, if any, can lend the subject clarity. This conversation begins with a consideration of the difference between good science and bad science.

THE PROBLEM OF CREATING GOOD SCIENCE

A general definition of *science* is the asking and answering of questions through a controlled process of testing, repeating, and confirming results. The scientific method we all learned in grade school covers the basic contours: to know if a thing is true, one must isolate that thing and test it without changing anything else. Change two or more things, and you introduce the possibility that your results might come from any or all of them; no definitive answers can emerge until the universe of possible explanations is winnowed down to a final candidate.

To deal with this problem in human studies, scientists usually create a comparison group alongside the group being tested—the *control group*. This group, as the name suggests, helps scientists control for factors that might be acting on the experiment from elsewhere, offering a simple way to tell if the results are due to the experiment or something else. Without a control group, it is dismayingly easy to produce a "finding" that cannot withstand further scrutiny. Say, for instance, the test group in a drug experiment develops a rash. One might assume that the drug causes the rash. But if the untreated control group develops the same rash, then it is most likely due to something unseen that's influencing both groups, and not the drug.

Human research tends to cleave into two major "kingdoms": observational studies and controlled studies. Observational studies *observe* and *compare* groups of people. This research is conducted passively; in other words, without interventions or controls. Any significant differences that emerge between the populations studied—say, finding that people who drink more diet soda tend to have a higher incidence of depression than people who don't—can't prove anything but may be used to generate hypotheses about what is causing this difference.

Yet people still assume the obvious when confronted with a correlation of this sort. In the diet soda study, which was actually run by the National Institute of Health and widely reported, many people jumped to the conclusion that depression must be caused by something in the soda.[1] But a moment of creative consideration turns up several other plausible possibilities. What if the people who drink diet soda are simply more judgmental about their body appearance and generally more prone to self-criticism? What if, since drinking more diet soda correlates with a history of being overweight, the depression arises physiologically from the effects of obesity, or as a result of the cluster of health problems that go along with it, such as obstructive sleep apnea and diabetes? What if people who are depressed simply crave sweet things, as evidence suggests? And what of the fact that diet soda drinkers tend to cluster more in urban areas: is there something about this environment that promotes depression?

Strong correlation is tantalizing, a just-so homily that satisfies our need for simple explanations. It feels definitive and self-apparent, especially given the huge number of subjects typically involved in such studies. The NIH study that produced the diet soda finding, for instance, had 260,000 subjects. Headlines are driven and public health advice administered whenever a major observational study unearths a provocative new correlation. But it turns out that the record of observational studies like these for generating accurate medical advice is, in a word, abysmal. Award-winning science journalist Gary Taubes described the issue in the *New York Times Magazine*:

Stephen Pauker, a professor of medicine at Tufts University and a pioneer in the field of clinical decision making, says, "Epidemiologic studies, like diagnostic tests, are probabilistic statements." They don't tell us what the truth is, he says, but they allow both physicians and patients to "estimate the truth" so they can make informed decisions. The question the skeptics will ask, however, is how can anyone judge the value of these studies without taking into account their track record? And if they take into account the track record, suggests Sander Greenland, an epidemiologist at the University of California, Los Angeles, and an author of the textbook "Modern Epidemiology," then wouldn't they do just as well if they simply tossed a coin?[2]

The only way to answer these questions would be to run a *randomized study*. This is a type of controlled study in which people are randomly assigned to respective groups—in this case, one group drinks diet soda, one drinks regular soda, one drinks a third option or no soda at all. Randomization eliminates any question about whether certain kinds of people self-select into certain groups. As Taubes relates:

> In January 2001, the British epidemiologists George Davey Smith and Shah Ebrahim, co-editors of *The International Journal of Epidemiology* . . . noted that those few times that a randomized trial had been financed to test a hypothesis supported by results from these large observational studies, the hypothesis either failed the test or, at the very least, the test failed to confirm the hypothesis: antioxidants like vitamins E and C and beta carotene did not prevent heart disease, nor did eating copious fiber protect against colon cancer.[3]

It is an intriguing question: why *do* purely observational studies fail so often despite finding such clear associations? The diet soda example tells the tale. All of those alternative theories I mentioned can be boiled down to a single, devastating possibility: what if diet soda drinkers are just *fundamentally different* from regular soda drinkers, in any of the ways I mentioned, and this difference colors *everything* about the way they live and behave? Scientists call this the *selection effect*, or *selection bias.* When human beings are free to behave as they always have—free to willfully choose their behavior—there is no meaningful way to find a control group of comparable subjects.

THE DEVIL IN COMPLIANCE

Selection bias has been widely studied, and today we are aware of many ways that this effect can despoil scientific studies. Yet one way deserves special mention, as it has threatened to undermine the very core of public health research: the *compliance effect.*

A growing body of evidence strongly suggests that people who do things faithfully and regularly for their own well-being, such as taking a multivitamin, exercising daily, or eating a certain diet, are, in fact, fundamentally different from people who don't. People who adhere to, or *comply with*, medical advice are more likely to take care of themselves in numerous other ways as well:

> Quite simply, people who comply with their doctors' orders when given a prescription are different and healthier than people who don't. This difference may be ultimately unquantifiable. The compliance effect is another plausible explanation for many of the beneficial associations that epidemiologists commonly report, which means this alone is a reason to wonder if much of what we hear about what constitutes a healthful diet and lifestyle is misconceived.[4]

The compliance effect can lead researchers and reporters who study interventions to falsely credit a pill or diet with improving our health— "Look, people who take fish oil pills live longer than the rest of us!"— when the truth may be far more subtle: the *kind* of people who take supplements in a disciplined way are already healthier to begin with, with a better prognosis for every disease.

This is another reason why large observational studies regularly fail when they are examined with better scientific controls. Pomegranate juice, red wine, and chocolate have all failed to show any appreciable health benefit once studied under controlled conditions. In the case of hormone replacement therapy, famously, it turned out that all those observational studies had it exactly backwards: the women who faithfully took hormone pills lived longer because they were the kind of women who were simply more attuned to their health, period. Chillingly, researchers later discovered that the pills were working *against* this natural advantage.

The funhouse mirror widens. The compliance effect has led to some famously strange epidemiological results. One long-term study showed that people who took a *placebo* were half as likely to die as those who did not. Was the placebo protecting them in some way the researchers had failed to anticipate? Hardly. It turned out that simply taking the placebo regularly was a signpost for a wholly different lifestyle. The pill takers were simply more actively engaged in their health across the board.

A poor understanding of these issues—the need for randomization, the difference between correlation and causation, and the power of the compliance effect—has colored much of the research that has been conducted to date about the effectiveness of 12-step membership and attendance. Other studies have been bedeviled by inadequate analysis of the data itself, including sloppy omissions and statistical errors. Deborah Dawson of the National Institute on Alcohol Abuse and Alcoholism, Division of Biometry and Epidemiology, once lamented the lack of credible data in the study of addiction treatment: "Few, if any, studies have assessed the impact of different types of treatment on both the probability and rapidity of recovery, i.e. on person-years of dependence averted."[5] Her principal complaint: the lack of controls in most AA studies.

WHAT IS SUCCESS?

Analyzing the available data about AA requires that we begin with a clear definition of success. *Success*, after all, can mean any number of things. Should one measure it in days of sobriety? Weeks without a binge episode? What if people who are making substantive progress slip and have one drink during an otherwise successful period of time: Should they "go back to zero," as is the practice in many AA chapters? What if they stop drinking but acquire a gambling problem instead?

The question of prognosis is far easier to answer in the rest of medicine. Disease is usually a binary system: either you've got it or you don't. Pneumonia: got it or you don't. HIV: got it or you don't. Multiple sclerosis, polio, emphysema—all of these are yes-or-no propositions. But alcoholism is not, in fact, a disease: it is a *behavior*, or perhaps a collection of behaviors. And because nobody can say for sure whether a behavior has ever been eliminated for good without a crystal ball, we must first establish a baseline definition of what success looks like in the treatment of addiction. I'll propose this simple definition:

> A treatment for alcoholism may be called successful if an individual no longer drinks in a way that is harmful in his or her life.

THE CLAIMS OF 12-STEP PROGRAMS

AA does not hew to a single company line on the question of its success rate; various accounts have quoted the organization as saying "upward of 75 percent of its members maintain abstinence."[6] Here, again, is that key passage I cited from *Alcoholics Anonymous*:

> Rarely have we seen a person fail who has thoroughly followed our path. Those who do not recover are people who cannot or will not completely give themselves to this simple program, usually men and women who are constitutionally incapable of being honest with themselves. There are such unfortunates. They are not at fault; they seem to have been born that way. They are naturally incapable of grasping and developing a manner of living which demands rigorous honesty. Their chances are less than average. There are those, too, who suffer from grave emotional and mental disorders, but many of them do recover if they have the capacity to be honest.[7]

To understand what can actually be known about AA's success rate, we must attempt a deep dive into the best data available. Let's start with the controlled studies.

At least one early attempt to study Alcoholics Anonymous in a randomized experiment was run by J. M. Brandsma (of the College of

Medicine at the University of Kentucky) and colleagues in 1980.[8] Eighty individuals, mainly court-referred, were randomized into three groups: AA-based treatment run by the investigators; a course of one-on-one RBT (rational behavioral therapy) run by lay people; and an open option for patients to choose any treatment they wished, which constituted a control group.

The investigators found "significantly more binge drinking at the 3-month follow-up" among the people assigned to the AA-oriented meetings. As the year mark approached, the researchers noted, "All of the lay-RBT clients reported drinking less during the last 3 months. This was significantly better than the AA or the control groups at the 0.005 level [meaning the finding was highly statistically significant]." The final data led the researchers to conclude: "In this analysis the AA group was five times more likely to binge than the control group and nine times more likely than the lay-RBT group. The AA group average was 2.4 binges in the last 3 months."

It was a provocative result, but hardly definitive. After all, a good scientist could imagine any number of factors that might have confounded the numbers in this study. The nature of the "lay therapy" is never well defined, for instance, nor were any measures taken to ensure that this option was provided in a uniform way. The "choice" group is never broken out into subsets that might allow us to see which treatments they chose, if any. And, like almost all longitudinal studies, this one relied on self-reporting, which is a notoriously questionable metric.

The results, however, did mirror what was concluded in later trials involving AA. A review of all such reports between 1976 and 1989 was performed by C. D. Emrick (of the School of Medicine of the University of Colorado) and colleagues. The researchers concluded:

> The effectiveness of AA as compared to other treatments for "alcoholism" has yet to be demonstrated. Reliable guidelines have not been established for predicting who among AA members will be successful. . . . Caution was raised against rigidly referring every alcohol-troubled person to AA.[9]

It took until 1991 for another randomized study to be completed. This one found essentially the same results as the Brandsma study. In a paper published in the *New England Journal of Medicine*, the oldest continuously published medical journal in the world and widely considered the world's most prestigious, D. C. Walsh and his co-researchers "randomly assigned a series of 227 workers newly identified as abusing alcohol to one of three rehabilitation regimens: compulsory inpatient treatment, compulsory attendance at AA meetings, and a choice of options. The findings were notable:

> On seven measures of drinking and drug use . . . we found significant differences at several follow-up assessments. The hospital group fared best and that assigned to AA the least well; those allowed to choose a program had intermediate outcomes. Additional inpatient treatment was required significantly more often . . . by the AA group (63 percent) and the choice group (38 percent) than by subjects assigned to initial treatment in the hospital (23 percent).[10]

These results led the researchers to issue a warning in their final recommendations: "An initial referral to AA alone or a choice of programs, although less costly than inpatient care, involves more risk than compulsory inpatient treatment and should be accompanied by close monitoring for signs of incipient relapse."

THE MOST MEASURED REVIEW

All scientists are aware of the dangers of non-controlled studies, of course, but often they have no choice. Randomizing individuals and controlling carefully for outside factors is extremely expensive, far more so than running an observational study. Controlled experiments can be conducted only with small sample sizes and with the help of deep pockets. As a result, proper clinical data is maddeningly hard to come by in many questions of public health.

Yet one group exists solely to sort through the glut of studies and help caregivers tune out poorly designed or reported research: the Cochrane Collaboration, which comprises nearly thirty thousand researchers dedicated to pushing back against what medical pioneer David Sacket once called "the disastrous inadequacy of lesser evidence."[11] The Collaboration's mission is quite simply to focus only on studies with proper protocols and minimal bias and to assemble the strongest data from a rigorously defined set of criteria. No purely observational studies or uncontrolled studies are permitted in a *Cochrane Review*; the organization's goal, simply put, is to vet all the science out there and tell us what can actually be verified.

In 2006, the Cochrane Collaboration undertook a characteristically careful and detailed look at studies of AA and 12-step recovery. First, the researchers recapped what had been determined to date:

> [A] meta-analysis [historic analysis of previous studies] by Kownacki (1999) identified severe selection bias in the available studies, with the randomised studies yielding worse results [for AA] than non-randomised studies. This meta-analysis is weakened by the heterogeneity of patients and interventions that are pooled together. Emrick 1989 performed a narrative review of studies about characteristics of alcohol-dependent individuals who affiliate with AA and concluded that the effectiveness of AA as compared to other treatments for alcoholism was not clear and therefore needed to be demonstrated.[12]

The Collaboration then identified eight high-quality, controlled, randomized studies, with 3,417 subjects in all.[13] Their conclusion was unambiguous: "No experimental studies unequivocally demonstrated the effectiveness of AA or TSF [Twelve Step Facilitation] approaches for reducing alcohol dependence or problems."

Despite the fact that the best designed studies have all questioned AA's effectiveness, there remains a body of academic articles that are very frequently cited by supporters of the 12-step movement. To understand the arguments of 12-step proponents, we must give these studies an open hearing as well.

In 1999, R. Fiorentine and colleagues ran a twenty-four-month lon-gitudinal after-treatment study that "suggests the effectiveness of 12-step programs." They concluded:

> the findings suggest that weekly or more frequent 12-step participa-tion is associated with drug and alcohol abstinence. Less-than-weekly participation is not associated with favorable drug and alcohol use out-comes, and participation in 12-step programs seems to be equally use-ful in maintaining abstinence from both illicit drug and alcohol use. These findings point to the wisdom of a general policy that recom-mends weekly or more frequent participation in a 12-step program as a useful and inexpensive aftercare resource for many clients.[14]

The authors of this paper based their recommendations on a clear correlation that has appeared many times in the literature, namely that the longer people attend AA meetings, the more likely they are to ex-perience better outcomes for sobriety. Here is how they summarized their findings:

> In the 6-month period prior to the 24-month follow-up, approxi-mately 27% of those participating in any 12-step meetings used an il-licit drug compared to 44% of those not attending 12-step meetings. The results of the urinalysis support the same conclusion. About 28% of those attending any 12-step meetings tested positive for an illicit drug at the 24-month follow-up compared to 41% of those not at-tending 12-step meetings. Less than 4% of 12-step participants tested positive for alcohol at the 24-month follow-up compared to about 13% of nonattendees.

In other words, the incidence of drinking was roughly 60 percent higher among nonattendees than attendees at the first two measure-ments and far higher at the final data point, to the tune of a 300 percent improvement for the AA attenders.

It's tempting to look at correlations like this and conclude, as many have, that AA must be responsible for this improvement. Yet Fiorentine and his colleagues themselves noted that their results were at odds with other recent studies like the Walsh study cited above and another by B. S. McCrady, who both found that "random assignment to AA or two other treatment condition groups did not reveal more-favorable drinking outcomes for AA participants."[15] The researchers were also mindful of the compliance effect:

> The findings suggest that 12-step programs may be an effective step in maintaining drug and alcohol abstinence. Unfortunately, the limitations of the design do not allow other variables, including the *motivational confound*, to be ruled out as possible influences on the drug and alcohol use outcomes of 12-step participants. (Emphasis added)

Hence their highly qualified final recommendation, which is not often cited by 12-step proponents:

> More definitive answers to these questions may come from randomized trials involving 12-step programs and comparison groups of sufficient size that are followed over a relatively long posttreatment duration. . . . Randomized designs are the best method yet to disaggregate the effectiveness of treatment from other influences, including motivational differences. . . . [T]he findings indicate that both weekly and less-than-weekly 12-step participants had very high recovery motivation scores—scores that may be attributable, at least in part, to the sampling bias of the study.

Caveats such as these are standard practice in peer-reviewed science, so they should be taken only as possibilities, not as an indictment of the research as a whole. Yet the significance of these warnings cannot be overstated: anyone who understands the inherent difficulties with observational science would recognize this list of concerns as grounds to consider the results provisional until a controlled study can be mounted.

Fiorentine and his colleagues did attempt to minimize the effects of sampling bias by doing what researchers almost always do in epidemiological science: they applied multiple regression analysis (MRA), which involves developing a mathematical model to try to explain the data, and to account for and separate out all the known differences between the groups—*disaggregate*, in their language. MRA unquestionably has its uses, but it can no more overlay controls retroactively on an uncontrolled study than a camera can turn a single still image into a 360-degree panorama. In elegant understatement, Harvard Medical School professor and epidemiologist Jerry Avorn told the *New York Times* that MRA "doesn't always work as well as we'd like it to."[16]

Indeed, what troubles many good scientists about research like the Fiorentine paper is that studying the people who *choose* to attend AA is an almost perfect recipe for generating the compliance effect error. AA members who frequently attend meetings may be demonstrating the same sort of self-care qualities that the placebo takers do. They may be, in effect, the Boy Scouts, or "eager patients," of the addict population.[17] Nobody who has looked at this data would dispute that people who attend AA most often and stay the longest are more likely to improve than the dropouts. The question is whether AA is driving this outcome or benefiting from a correlation instead.

Is it possible that the kind of people who stay in 12-step programs are *already* more likely to improve? Would they be equally likely to do so in any treatment, or even no treatment at all? At heart, the dilemma facing AA research is whether people stay in AA because they're the type of people who will stick with a program no matter what it is and who would have stuck with it even if it were of no help to them at all.

THE MOOS DATA

In 2005, husband-and-wife team Rudolph and Bernice Moos of Stanford University published the first of two papers that would become some of the most-cited data in support of Alcoholics Anonymous.[18] Because these articles have become major sources of faith in the effectiveness of AA, they deserve an especially careful review.

The authors conducted a longitudinal, observational study of 362 previously untreated people who chose to enter either AA, professional treatment, or a combination of both. Notably, the authors never defined what was meant by "professional treatment," or the level of training or competence of the professionals performing the treatment, a point they conceded in the 2006 paper, "Participation in Treatment and Alcoholics Anonymous": "[An] issue involves the lack of data on the content of treatment, which might have enabled us to examine whether aspects of psychological and social functioning changed less because they were not addressed adequately in treatment."

In truth, the word *treatment* could mean almost anything in this context, including the very real possibility that it was 12-step-based as well, or was "motivational enhancement therapy," which is a brief encouragement-based approach that does not resemble serious psychotherapy. The paper's definition of "long-term treatment" is also mistaken. The researchers defined this as anything more than six months, while most well-trained and experienced professionals in psychology would consider that a short-term treatment.

Surveys were sent out at various checkpoints: one, three, eight, and sixteen years. In their first paper, the researchers concluded:

> Compared with individuals who participated only in professional treatment in the first year after they initiated help-seeking, individuals who participated in both [professional] treatment and AA were more likely to achieve remission. Individuals who entered treatment but delayed participation in AA did not appear to obtain any additional benefit from AA.[19]

It was, in other words, a mixed bag. Visit a therapist and AA together, the data suggests, and you are likely to do better than you would with therapy alone. But visit a therapist for one year and *then* try AA, and you won't do any better than if you had just stayed in therapy.

Notably, the researchers went on to publish a far more strongly worded follow-up in 2006, drawing from the same data. This paper begins by demonstrating some similarities in compliance with treatment between the AA attendees and "treatment" group:

> In the first year . . . 273 (59.2%) of the 461 individuals entered professional treatment and 269 (58.4%) entered AA. In the second and third

years of follow-up, 167 individuals (36.2%) were in treatment and 176 (38.2%) participated in AA. In years 4 to 8, 144 individuals (31.2%) were in treatment and 166 (36.0%) participated in AA.[20]

Unsurprisingly, they found that the people who stuck with *either* treatment—AA or professional treatment—did significantly better than those who did not. These were the compliers. The authors continue:

> Compared with individuals who remained untreated, individuals who obtained 27 weeks or more of treatment in the first year after seeking help had better 16-year alcohol-related outcomes. Similarly, individuals who participated in AA for 27 weeks or more had better 16-year outcomes. Subsequent AA involvement was also associated with better 16-year outcomes, but this was not true of subsequent treatment.[21]

In other words, again unsurprisingly, they found that the people who stuck with either approach—AA or professional treatment—did significantly better than those who did not. Yet the last sentence suggests that people continued to improve over time with AA, whereas they failed to continue improving with treatment. (The authors measured improvement via self-reports in answer to questions such as "Have you been sad the past month?" or "Have you participated in social activities?") What their conclusion doesn't address, however, is the possibility that the people in treatment were *already* doing better than the AA group, and that they therefore had less room to improve over those last eight years. We do not know, nor do the researchers say, which interpretation is right.

More problematic is that the study elided some potentially telling fluctuations in the data. People who stayed in AA for fewer than six months had *worse* outcomes than people who never entered AA at all. This finding seems to mirror the Brandsma data: AA attendees seem to get worse before they get better. One theory is that the finding is nothing but *noise*—the standard statistical turbulence that can foul any short-term study. But if the data are real and repeatable, then they suggest something the Moos researchers perhaps did not consider: that AA might do more harm than good for the people who *choose* to attend but do not *buy into* the program.

The Moos study also employs some objectionable statistical methods. In one critical omission, its conclusions ignore all the people who died and the large number of people who dropped out of the study altogether, despite conceding that these were the people who statistically consumed the most alcohol. As early as year eight, the number of subjects who were left in AA had already shrunk by nearly 40 percent (from 269 to 166), yet these people are erased from the conclusions as if they had never existed at all. Add up all the people who died and the dropouts, and the results for AA become far grimmer than the authors suggest.

The stated size of this survey is also misleading. Although the researchers began with 628 people, the total number of people who remained through the sixteen-year follow-up *and* also stayed in AA for longer than six months—that is, the group on which the authors' major findings are based—was just 107, or 17 percent of the original sample. And of the remaining 107, the researchers never revealed the actual number of people who improved, or even stayed sober. They told us only which group "had better outcomes."

Next, there is the question of validity of the results. As I have mentioned, self-reporting is a tricky methodology, prone to the illusions of self-deception and imperfect memory. In most observational research, surveys are the standard currency—without surveys, there can be no data. Yet there are ways to mitigate the information people report about themselves, notably independent testing. The Moos study did not attempt to independently verify any of the surveys it was based on. (The Fiorentine group, by contrast, supplemented their surveys with urine tests.)

Finally, the punctuated nature of the study addressed only the six-month windows prior to each of the four check-ins. This meant that of the sixteen years covered by the study, the researchers' surveys gathered information on only two of them. No questions were ever asked about the stretches of time in between follow-ups; 88 percent of the time was never studied. As the authors acknowledged in the 2006 paper, "Another limitation is that we obtained information only on 6-month windows of alcohol-related outcomes at each follow-up, and thus cannot trace the complete drinking status of respondents over the 16-year interval."

Ultimately none of these issues should be great enough to disqualify the Moos study on its own. But together they should give us pause. The study had no controls, so subjects were free to join and leave treatment as they wished. And for every slice of subjects that got better, the study omitted many about which we are never told a thing. Possibly as a consequence of these limitations, the authors of the study readily acknowledged that they, too, struggled with the question of cause and effect:

> [I]ndividuals self-selected into treatment and AA and, based on their experiences, decided on the duration of participation. Thus, in part, the benefits we identified are due to the influence of self-selection and motivation to obtain help as well as that of longer participation per se. Although our findings probably reflect the real-world effectiveness of participation in treatment and AA for alcohol use disorders, the naturalistic design precludes firm inferences about the causal role of treatment or AA.

A BIG QUESTION

Why do large observational studies such as that of Fiorentine and Moos seem to suggest that AA is effective, while smaller controlled studies like those of the Brandsma, Walsh, and others included in the *Cochrane Review* do not? The likely explanation is simple: people stay in AA if they're getting better and leave if they aren't. This is understandable. If you are able to stop drinking, then continuing to attend AA is a comfortable and affirming choice. If you struggle with drinking and can't make use of the AA approach, then you are less likely to keep attending. Over the long term, the people who remain in AA are, by definition, the success stories. But they represent a very small slice of the people who start there; as we will see shortly, the dropout rate from AA is extremely high.

These facts—that AA works for the diehards and fails for the dropouts—are perennially misunderstood by the press and even by some researchers. Proponents of the program proudly point to the fact that people who stay in AA tend to be sober, ignoring the tautological nature of this claim. Reviewing this logic, Harvard biostatistics professor Richard Gelber said, "The main problem is the self-fulfilling prophesy: the longer people stick with AA the better they are, hence AA must be working. It is like saying the longer you live, the older you will be when you die." As we will soon see, this fundamental error in logic undergirds nearly every claim of AA's efficacy.

Despite the known limitations with the Moos data set, a number of researchers have used it to publish pro-AA papers of their own. For instance, in 2008, J. McKellar (writing as lead author, with Ilgen, Moos, and Moos as coauthors) concluded that "clinicians should focus on keeping patients engaged in AA."[22] This recommendation is even more dogmatic than Moos and Moos suggested in their original paper. In fact, this paper itself notes that pressuring people to attend AA is usually unhelpful: "a significant number of substance abuse patients never attend self-help groups after discharge," that is, when no longer mandated to attend.

In 2011, again, using the original Moos data, Stanford's Christine Timko published as lead author on another paper with Moos and Moos, drawing a similar conclusion:

> Among initially untreated individuals, sustained mutual help may be associated with a reduced number of occurrences of DWI [Driving While Intoxicated arrests] via fewer drinking consequences and improved psychological functioning and coping. Treatment providers should attend to these concomitants of DWI and consider actively referring individuals to AA to ensure ongoing AA affiliation.[23]

Another observational AA study was conducted by John-Kåre Vederhus in 2006, once again without randomization or any interventions. This one looked at a small group—just 114 patients—with drug and alcohol problems, and found the same broad correlation as Moos and Moos: Intention-to-treat-analysis showed that 38 percent still participated in self-help programs two years after treatment. Among the regular participants, 81 percent had been abstinent over the previous 6 months, compared with only 26 percent of the non-participants.[24]

Once again, after two years, over 60 percent of the people remaining in the study had dropped out of AA. The people who stayed were admirably sober, on the order of 81 percent. But the total number of people who were sober and still attending AA was only 31 percent of the whole group. Despite this figure, and despite the fact that the study involved only people who had self-selected into 12-step programs and that nearly 35 percent of subjects had dropped out entirely, biasing the results toward more positive outcomes, the authors state, "We conclude that the probability of a positive effect is sufficient to recommend participation in self-help groups as a supplement to drug addiction treatment." This study was repeated in our popular press as proof positive that AA was a success.

In 2012, yet another longitudinal and observational study, conducted in Sacramento, California, by Jane Witbrodt and colleagues, found essentially the same results as the prior studies, namely, that the people who are still in AA at the end of many years tend to be admirably sober and well.[25] Once again, however, there were familiar issues: 25 percent of the study subjects had dropped out by year 9, and of those remaining, only 25 percent were "high" attenders of AA, which was the group with the best outcomes. (Even within this high-attending group, 22 percent were still drinking.) Like its cousins, this study relied on self-reporting and, like its cousins, acknowledged a major caveat: "We suspect that the higher abstinence in our 'high' class may be due in part to this being a more stably insured or employed population." The authors also acknowledged that they "lacked baseline measures for prior 12-step involvement and treatment episodes. Undoubtedly, these prior exposures may have influenced subsequent attendance for some study participants." It appears from this acknowledgment that the authors were aware that there was a pro-AA bias in the selection of their sample.

In fact, every one of the subjects in this paper had already been through the eight-week Chemical Dependency Recovery Program at the Kaiser Permanente facility in Sacramento, which is a 12-step-based program. In other words, all of the subjects of this study had already been exposed to the AA philosophy and actively encouraged to attend before they were followed up to determine if AA treatment would be helpful. It would be hard to imagine a clearer example of selection bias. If the authors had titled their article "Abstinence among People Intensively Exposed to AA Doctrine Who Then Chose to Continue with AA," they would have been on more solid ground.

The authors did, however, acknowledge that the big question was whether AA was helping people or not. To this point, they added a familiar caveat:

> Still, the direct relationship between 12-step attendance and abstinence remains uncertain in part because randomized clinical trials that direct and restrict attendance are difficult to conduct with such a freely available source of support as AA (and NA/CA). This relationship becomes even more blurred when attendance is studied over longer follow-up periods and as people transition in and out of both formal treatment programs and 12-step groups. In addition, only scant research has focused on outcomes other than actual alcohol and drug use (e.g., abstention status, percent days abstinent, drinks per drinking day).

Like the Moos and Fiorentine researchers before them, the Witbrodt researchers failed to address the simple fact that one cannot prove that any medical intervention works without a control group. (Interestingly the real "control" group for Alcoholics Anonymous—people who seek no treatment at all—have their own impressive rate of recovery, which I will discuss shortly.)

One paper has tried to tackle the question of whether we can determine causality in a direct way. A 2003 study, conducted by J. McKellar and colleagues of the Palo Alto Health Care System and published in the *Journal of Consulting and Clinical Psychology*, attempted to do a difficult thing—determine causality retroactively using statistical techniques and a method of multivariate analysis known as *structural modeling*, an approach that attempts to develop mathematical equations to explain existing data.[26] Such techniques are not uncommon in medicine, although doubts about their value persist. After a good deal of mathematical fireworks, the study's authors determined that AA attendance was associated with a reduction in alcohol-related problems, but that reduced alcohol-related problems were not associated with AA attendance. In other words, AA attendance actually *caused* a reduction in alcohol-related problems, rather than simply correlating with them.

Yet a closer look at the paper's methodology raises some important questions about both the model and the generalizability of its findings. The researchers didn't look at a representative sample of the general population. The study was populated by mostly (86 percent) single men, all of whom were veterans and all of whom had been in a 12-step in-patient program previously and were subsequently referred to AA. There were no controls or randomization. About one-quarter of all study participants dropped out and were not considered in the paper's conclusions.

This study's findings hewed fairly closely to what we've seen before: at one-year follow-up, hazardous consumption decreased from 93 percent to 42 percent, and decreased further to 37.5 percent at two years (a further 10.7 percent drop); at the same one-year follow-up, 80 percent of the subjects were involved with AA (an increase of 24 percent over baseline). At two years, 68 percent were still involved.

Yet these numbers, which suggest a strong correlation between AA attendance and sobriety, become less impressive when one looks more closely at the results. After one year, for instance, hazardous use dropped about 50 percent even though AA involvement increased by only 24 percent. It would therefore be difficult to attribute this improvement to AA alone. Far more likely is the possibility that a series of other factors lent a helping hand, including the hospitalization itself. Even *intensive* AA involvement—the kind most associated with better outcomes among AA members—during that first year was reported to be up by just 14 percentage points (from 9.2 percent to 23.3 percent) despite the 50 percent improvement, suggesting again that the improvement may have had to do with factors beyond AA. (More on this in a moment.)

The key point is a statistical one. When AA involvement and better outcomes move in the same direction, even if they are out of proportion, that represents a plausible correlation that might indeed turn out to be a causal relationship. On the other hand, when the numbers move in *opposite* directions, that is considered a clear negative result. This is precisely what happened in the first two years of the McKellar study. The paper reports that AA involvement decreased by 12 percent, while "hazardous" drinking went down by 11 percent. (The authors defined hazardous drinking as consuming more than four drinks on a drinking day.) This is the reverse of what one would expect if AA were responsible for the improvement: as people dropped out of AA, drinking should have become worse, not better.

As Harvard biostatistician Richard Gelber notes,

> That both alcohol-related problems and participation in AA seemed to decline between years 1 and 2 by the same amount raises questions about the conclusion from the structural modeling used. It does not pass the common sense test. . . . This direct evidence calls into question conclusions drawn from the structural modeling.[27]

Of course, the demographic issue alone, including the fact that everyone in the study had already been through 12-step treatment before, disqualifies this paper as a representative look at what happens when a cross-section of alcoholics is treated. McKellar and colleagues themselves noted, "Because individuals were not randomly assigned to attend self-help groups, one could argue that the apparently positive outcomes are due to self-selection on prognostic variables other than those we tested, such as available social support or willingness to self-disclose."[28]

As with other studies, the McKellar researchers also took no steps to verify the self-reported data about drinking frequency, either through urine tests or check-ins with friends or relatives. Ultimately, the authors acknowledged that the study failed to answer some very basic questions:

> Future studies comparing AA with other interventions might help answer important questions such as (a) Does AA provide specialized benefits in lowering long-term alcohol problems when compared with other self-help groups or outpatient after care programs? or conversely; (b) Does AA affiliation (attending meeting, working the steps, etc.) provide the same benefits that any good therapeutic treatment would

provide (i.e., hope, treatment rationale, therapeutic alliance, mitigation of isolation; Bergin & Garfield, 1994)?

Remarkably, despite all this, the McKellar study authors concluded that "the findings are consistent with the hypothesis that AA participation has a positive effect on alcohol-related outcomes."

THE MOTIVATION QUESTION

A recurring theme in AA research is the question of what *kind* of people do well in AA. Is there something about this small group of people, some special stuff, that makes them different? And if so, can we possibly ascertain what that stuff is? One paper, published by L. A. Kaskutas and colleagues of the School of Public Health, University of California, Berkeley, in 2009, took a look at the existing data and found, as the Cochrane Collaboration did, a lack of solid grounding for the claim that AA is a cure for alcoholism or addiction:

> Rigorous experimental evidence establishing the specificity of an effect for AA or Twelve Step Facilitation/TSF (criteria 5) is mixed, with 2 trials finding a positive effect for AA, 1 trial finding a negative effect for AA, and 1 trial finding a null effect. Studies addressing specificity using statistical approaches have had two contradictory findings, and two that reported significant effects for AA after adjusting for potential confounders such as motivation to change.[29]

This mix of results squares with what we have seen thus far in this chapter. The strong evidence that one would expect if AA were clearly effective is simply not present. At best, the proponents of the 12-step model can claim only what AA claims; namely, that the program "works if you work it." Which is another way of saying that people who do well, do well. What does this mean about whether AA itself "works"?

In 2005, R. D. Weiss and colleagues at Harvard Medical School conducted a study that looked more closely at what drives people to a higher level of success in 12-step programs. In the study, which randomized 487 cocaine-dependent outpatients to various twenty-four-week behavioral treatments, the authors uncovered a strong indication that attendance alone did not seem to help people with addictions, but that "*active* 12-step participation" was predictive: "Twelve-step group attendance did not predict subsequent drug use. However, active 12-step participation in a given month predicted less cocaine use in the next month."[30]

In 2011, J. Majer of Harry S. Truman College in Chicago and colleagues completed a longitudinal study of people in sober houses and reached much the same conclusion:

> Participants who were "categorically involved" in all 12-step [recommended] activities [having a sponsor, reading 12-step literature, doing service work, and calling other members for help] reported significantly higher levels of abstinence and self-efficacy for abstinence at 1 year compared with those who were less involved, whereas averaged summary scores of involvement were not a significant predictor of abstinence.[31]

Here it was again: evidence that more *engagement* with the program was correlated with greater abstinence (even though more *attendance* was not). The Weiss and Majer studies together suggest that the helpful factor in AA treatment may be the level of engagement or sense of group membership, rather than the therapeutic value of the meetings themselves. Of course this interpretation, too, might just be backward: it is entirely possible that the people who do well in AA become more involved as a result—that is, sobriety drives participation.

By now, the danger of looking at such correlations and concluding that people with alcoholism should go to AA should be evident. It would be akin to recommending that therapists try to get people into religion if they believe religious people are more contented. People who are devout have self-selected into religious organizations because this is meaningful to them. But that devotion cannot be imposed on others. People who do well in AA might very well self-select because they find it meaningful for some reasons I will describe later in this book. But given the results of all the studies on 12-step treatment, trying to push others into AA, who are less likely to find it meaningful, is a mistake.

The practice of recommending AA to all problem drinkers may also be harmful, as suggested by evidence that AA dropouts do worse than those who seek no treatment at all. The Moos study, for example, found that people who attended but did not stick with AA had worse outcomes than people who never entered the program. This makes sense, since failing to benefit from the approach that others claim to be the best (or only) effective treatment is depressing indeed. Often this depression is exacerbated when the person is blamed for not adequately "working" the program.

ACTUAL NUMBERS

Even though AA does not conduct scientific studies on its success rates, a number of clinicians have tried to audit the figures. The National Longitudinal Alcohol Epidemiologic Survey, a 1992 review by the US Census Bureau and National Institute on Alcohol Abuse and Alcoholism (NIAAA), included a survey of AA members. It found that only 31 percent of them were still attending after one year.[32] AA itself has published a comparable figure in a set of comments on its own thirteen-year internal survey, stating that only 26 percent of people who attend AA stay for longer than one year.[33] A third study found that after eighteen months, between 14 and 18 percent of people still attended AA.[34] So let us assume that between 14 percent and 31 percent of people stay with AA for more than one year. Now we must ask: out of this remaining population, how many stay sober?

As we have seen, research has shown that only a small subset of people stay sober in AA for any appreciable length of time, and this subset grows smaller with each passing year. When people do attend AA often or regularly, especially when they become emotionally invested in the system ("AA involvement" as opposed to "AA attendance," as the literature describes), they do well. As noted above, attending a self-help program per se is not helpful, but the *active* involvement seems to make a difference.

So, what percentage of AA attendees become actively involved? In 2003, a group in London headed by J. Harris looked at patients in residential treatment and concluded that while 75 percent of alcoholics entering residential treatment had attended AA previously, the number of those "working" the program (being "involved" versus merely attending) was 16/75, or 21 percent.[35]

Within this group, how many not only improved, but consistently maintained sobriety? University of California professor Herbert Fingarette cited two other statistics: at eighteen months, 25 percent of people still attended AA, and of those who did attend, 22 percent consistently maintained sobriety.[36] Taken together, these numbers show that about 5.5 percent of all those who started with AA became sober members. Similarly, taking the 21 percent "involved" from the Harris study and multiplying that by the 25 percent who remain in AA yields an overall efficacy of 5.25 percent. Or, we could use the more positive results of the Fiorentine study, in which "approximately 40 percent of individuals categorized as having continued active participation in AA maintained high rates of abstinence."[37] Combining this with the Harris data giving the percentage of people who are actively involved, overall effectiveness of AA becomes 21 percent times 40 percent, or 8.4 percent.

These totals all fall within a close range. Together, they support the fact that roughly 5 to 8 percent of the total population of people who enter AA are able to achieve and maintain sobriety for longer than one year.

THE PROBLEM OF SPONTANEOUS REMISSION

There is another issue that gets tangled up with the question of AA's success rate; namely, that a certain percentage of alcoholics get better without any treatment at all. This percentage is sometimes called the rate of *spontaneous remission*, a phrase commonly used in the world of oncology.

It is important to include spontaneous remission in any calculation of treatment efficacy, as it offers a more accurate baseline. It can also help to reveal the error in putative "cures" that are, on closer inspection, doing nothing at all. If one is trying to determine whether a certain drug can reverse arthritis, for instance, it's not enough to point out that 13 to 55 percent of people presenting with undifferentiated arthritis experienced a regression of the disease when given the drug: undifferentiated arthritis reverses on its own at precisely that rate.[38]

Different diagnoses have different degrees of spontaneous remission. In pancreatic cancer, spontaneous remission is unusual. For colds and flus, spontaneous remission is the norm. The burden of proof for any "cure" is to show that it clearly exceeds the rate of spontaneous remission for the targeted illness. If a treatment cannot perform better than doing nothing, it is likely that any apparent benefit is simply the phenomenon of spontaneous remission at work. Statistically speaking, it's background noise.

So what is the rate of spontaneous remission for alcoholism? One large study calculated it to be somewhere between 3.7 and 7.4 percent per year.[39] That is, in a given year, between 3.7 and 7.4 percent of alcoholics are likely to stop drinking without any help at all. A large 1990 meta-analysis by Sheldon Zimburg of the Beth Israel Medical Center in New York reviewed the available data about this and summarized the results:

> Kissin, Platz, and Su . . . reported a 4 percent one-year improvement rate in untreated lower class alcoholics. Imber et al. . . . . described a follow-up of 58 alcoholics who received no treatment for their alcoholism. It was noted that the rate of abstinence was 15 percent at one year and 11 percent after three years. . . . In sum, the preponderance of these studies suggests that a spontaneous remission rate for alcoholism of at least one-year duration is about 4–18 percent. Successful treatment would, therefore, have to produce rates of improvement significantly above this probable range of spontaneous remission.[40]

Could it be that some of AA's own modest success rate is attributable to spontaneous remission? Studies seem to support this idea. For instance, one controlled study from 2001 in Germany left patients free to choose AA treatment or no treatment at all. After one year, relapse rates were identical between the groups, leading the authors to conclude, "The present study was unable to show an advantage of self-help group attendance in reducing relapses compared to the control group [no treatment]."[41] Even one of AA's own board members, Harvard's George Vaillant, conducting an unusually long follow-up of his own AA-based hospital program, found "compelling evidence that the results of our treatment were no better than the natural history of the disease."[42]

PROJECT MATCH

In the late 1990s, one of the most ambitious studies ever undertaken to assess 12-step treatment was conducted. Called Project MATCH, it was underwritten by the National Institute on Alcohol Abuse and Alcoholism and funded to the tune of $27 million. Its stated goal was to determine which kind of treatment was best suited to which "kind" of alcoholics. The research showed a surprising finding, which has by now become an important statement about the power and frequency of spontaneous remission in alcoholism:

> Overall, a median of only 3% of the drinking outcome at follow-up could be attributed to treatment. However this effect appeared to be present at week one before most of the treatment had been delivered. The zero treatment dropout group showed great improvement, achieving a mean of 72 percent days abstinent at follow-up. Effect size estimates showed that two-thirds to three-fourths of the improvement in the full treatment group was duplicated in the zero treatment group.[43]

In 2005, Deborah Dawson and colleagues conducted a survey of 4,422 men to determine how many people classified as alcohol dependent remained that way in the absence of treatment.[44] They found a similar trend toward natural recovery:

> Of people classified with [prior] alcohol dependence, 25.0% were still classified as dependent in the past year; 27.3% were classified as being in partial remission; 11.8% were asymptomatic risk drinkers who demonstrated a pattern of drinking that put them at risk of relapse; 17.7% were low-risk drinkers; and 18.2% were abstainers. Only 25.5% of people with [prior] dependence ever received treatment.

In other words, about 36 percent of alcohol-dependent people in a general population study had become either low-risk drinkers or abstinent at the one-year mark, even though only 25.5 percent had received any treatment. It is worth noting that these were very serious drinkers, classified under the DSM criteria for "dependence," which requires not only a history of alcohol abuse but also physical dependence.

A FINAL WORD

Many claim that Alcoholics Anonymous is the only safe, effective, and consistent cure for alcoholism. Narcotics Anonymous, Gamblers Anonymous, and other 12-step offshoots enjoy a similar reputation for the treatment of their respective behaviors. Celebrity doctor Drew Pinsky ("Dr. Drew"), often described as an addiction medicine specialist and the host of VH1's *Celebrity Rehab*, once told *Wired* magazine, "In my 20 years of treating addicts, I've never seen anything else that comes close to the 12 steps. In my world, if someone says they don't want to do the 12 steps, I know they aren't going to get better."[45]

But, as we have seen, this unadulterated enthusiasm is quite simply unfounded. Most studies of AA that purport to show its effectiveness are observational in nature, with no controls that might help us capably determine results. They consistently point only to a correlation no one could debate; namely, that AA works well for the people who are the most invested in it. But this correlation becomes considerably less impressive when it is placed in the context of all the people who try but fail to benefit from 12-step recovery. An objective calculation puts AA's success rate at 5 to 8 percent. Controlled, randomized studies, on the other hand, have revealed an even more discouraging picture: no such study to date has been able to prove that AA is effective at all.

The issue of spontaneous remission further erodes AA's reputation. If alcoholism were something that people never recovered from on their own, then the 5–8 percent figure would be a small but meaningful slice of those with alcoholism in the general population. But many people do get better without treatment. In fact, as we've seen, a higher percentage of alcoholics get better without any treatment than with AA, suggesting that some of AA's success rate may simply be nature taking its course. There is also evidence that some people do worse by attending AA, as indicated in the McKellar results and in the experience of many who have foundered for years in AA before seeking more appropriate treatment (I will return to this later).

All that said, there is no question that AA is useful for some people. Some of this is due to characteristics that it shares with all collective organizations, such as camaraderie and support, as we will see later. In a later chapter, I will also explore some of the other factors that can help us understand AA through the prism of a more sophisticated understanding of the nature of addiction. Before we can get to that discussion, however, we must explore the industry Dr. Drew most strongly endorses. What about rehab?

CHAPTER FOUR

THE BUSINESS OF REHAB AND THE BROKEN PROMISE OF "AA-PLUS"

"The great thing about the Steps is they can be incorporated in so many facets of our lives, and working the Steps day after day makes us even better at it, too. The other great thing about the Steps is that they work. If they didn't work, then doing them over and over again would be insanity."

—BETTY FORD CENTER WEBSITE

THE ERA OF THE modern American addiction rehabilitation center officially began in 1949, when Hazelden Treatment Center opened its doors in Minnesota. Hazelden took the dictates of Alcoholics Anonymous and turned them into an inpatient model. It promised visitors and patients immersion in a version of the popular program that was more refined, without the interruptions present in regular 12-step meetings. It was, in a very real sense, an extension of AA into the twenty-four-hour day. Today, Hazelden still says that its program is "grounded in Twelve Step philosophy."[1] (Notably, although Hazelden also lists remaining "open to innovation" as a value, it has apparently not found ideas worthy of replacing the Twelve Steps over the past sixty-five years.)

Hazelden quickly became a tremendous financial and cultural success. Today, it commands fees in the range of $30,000 for a one-month stay. Its impact emboldened similar rehab centers to open across the nation, with a notable boom in the 1980s that birthed famous entries like the Betty Ford Center (1982) and Sierra Tucson (1983). As it happened, there was a large ready-made market for these programs, since millions of people were failing to stay sober in AA. The new "Cadillac" rehabs offered alcoholics a way to double down on the 12-step model—trying more, not less, of the same approach with which they were struggling.

This was a seductive idea that felt entirely consonant with the theme of spiritual cleansing and purity, and it rekindled the hope first created by Alcoholics Anonymous.

Almost immediately, a fierce competition began among the major rehab programs to add more and more "enhancements" to their treatment. Sure, these features added more cost, but what the programs were offering was practically priceless. Who would not be willing to spend a small fortune for a life free of the agony of addiction? For many addicts, the only question became: where to spend that fortune?

Sierra Tucson quickly developed what it calls the Sierra Model, which includes education about the disease model, recovery education, relapse prevention, "equine-assisted therapy," "adventure therapy," grief and spirituality sessions, and psychodrama. The Betty Ford Center has added meditation, fitness, educational lectures, relapse-prevention group, and therapeutic duty assignments. Hazelden offers, among other things, meditation, educational lectures, leisure skills groups, anger groups, stress management groups, relaxation, exercise, recreational activities, and biofeedback.

Rehabs also became increasingly opulent to compete for clientele. Playing into the idea that alcoholics needed a tranquil and beatific place to contemplate their problem or achieve spiritual fulfillment, many programs began to market themselves as spas. Betty Ford notes that its twenty-acre gated campus is "surrounded by serene mountains" and patients are housed in "spacious, double occupancy rooms."[2] Sierra Tucson boasts that its 160-acre campus sits in the shadow of the Santa Catalina Mountains; patients can move into "rustic and elegant lodges with cozy fireplaces, high beamed ceilings, outdoor balconies and patios."[3] The Menninger Clinic, previously justly famous as a psychiatric center, moved into the rehab business and released a flyer promising "outdoor terraces for each unit and a meditation labyrinth in the expansive courtyard."[4] And Promises Malibu, well-known redoubt of many A-list celebrities, entices its potential clients with descriptions like this:

> The property includes a garden, swimming pools, Jacuzzis, a tennis court, and numerous meditation areas for quiet reflection. Sun streams

through the beautifully decorated residences, bringing a feeling of warmth and healing comfort to the private rooms and common areas. With the mountains and ocean in your backyard, there are countless opportunities for outdoor, experiential activities including rock climbing and hiking. The beauty of the natural surroundings inspires a sense of awe and gratitude that encourages the recovery process.

Inside the facility, guests will be treated to gourmet meals, a fireplace, phone and internet access, and numerous patios and sitting areas.[5]

Today, as a result of this aggressive marketing, and helped along by a credulous media, rehab centers enjoy a reputation as the ultimate facilities for the treatment of addiction, the biggest and most comprehensive solutions the human mind can imagine. Hit TV shows like *Celebrity Rehab* and *Intervention* further the cause by continually preaching the gospel of rehab, often subtly equating "success" with mere admission. "Going to rehab" appears regularly in music and film as the ultimate hope for treating addiction.

Yet a surprisingly small number of these people have asked: *Is this industry actually helping people?* In this chapter I'll attempt to answer this question, beginning with an overview of the ways that rehab is both like, and unlike, Alcoholics Anonymous and other 12-step programs.

REHABS AND AA

Most rehab programs that borrow their philosophy from AA do so explicitly and do not attempt to hide their affiliation. If anything, it is generally a badge of pride within the rehab community that their methods have been adapted from a model that is widely seen as the best addiction treatment in the world. According to Hazelden's website, "The 'Minnesota Model' [is a] Twelve Step facilitation model [that] utilizes the philosophy of Alcoholics Anonymous as a therapeutic tool for recovery from addiction." Betty Ford informs us, "All our programs are based on the 12-steps of Alcoholics Anonymous," adding, "If, with courage and with total truth, you take the steps with absolutely no reservation, and eliminate those things from your life which, in good conscience, can't be reconciled with living the steps, you will stay sober." Sierra Tucson describes the Sierra Model as reflecting "a deep commitment to treating the whole person with integrated, individualized psychiatric and non-traditional therapies rooted in the Twelve-Step recovery process." The Kaiser Permanente Chemical Dependency Recovery Program that I mentioned in chapter 3 requires two 12-step meetings in the community each week plus an on-site 12-step meeting, and says that the 12-step philosophy is incorporated into some of its group sessions.

Of course there are some treatment centers that are explicitly non-disease-model and non-12-step. New York's St. Jude Retreats describes itself this way:

> First and foremost we are an alternative to traditional alcohol rehabs which means that we do not teach the disease concept of addiction (which has been proven in countless studies to be patently false for more than seventy years), we do not tell our guests they should feel guilty for their problems, and most importantly we do not tell people they will be in recovery for the rest of their lives. Saint Jude Retreats was the first non-disease based and non 12-step based program in America. We are working hard to educate individuals on the importance of knowing that addiction is and never will be a legitimate disease.[6]

However, St. Jude's is an outlier in this regard (and the program is unfortunately limited by employing a purely educational model, staffed by teachers rather than therapists).

Nearly all other rehab programs have some allegiance to the 12-step method. Even somewhat more psychologically sophisticated programs, such as Promises in California and the Fernside Center in Massachusetts, still incorporate the Twelve Steps into their philosophy.

All this begs the question: given that virtually every rehab is an elaborate expansion of 12-step meetings, why do people spend a fortune for programs that aren't fundamentally different from what they could find for free in a church basement?

THE ROLE OF HOSPITALIZATION

The biggest difference between rehabs and AA meetings on the outside is, of course, the element of institutionalization itself: being away from one's ordinary life while receiving constant care and support is a qualitatively separate experience from attending meetings from home.

Yet hospitalization isn't necessarily an unqualified good, nor is it considered "better" than outpatient treatment for many problems. In medicine, hospitalization is usually indicated only according to a specific set of criteria: patients are either unable to care for themselves, in precarious health, or in need of significant further treatment unavailable on the outside. No such criteria are applied at most of the biggest rehab centers, where admission decisions are generally made according to subjective and opaque processes, including, predominantly, the desire to be admitted and, of course, the ability to pay.

The duration of residence is treated differently in rehab than it is in either psychiatry or the rest of medicine as well. Nearly all credentialed medical facilities determine the length of a patient's stay according to that patient's diagnosis, history, and medical needs. Yet virtually every major rehabilitation center requires a lump-sum stay of twenty-eight, or sometimes thirty, days. (Promises Malibu opts for thirty, because "we want our clients to leave here with 30 days of sobriety," according to CEO David Sack.)[7] This number is applied without any special consideration of the health or prognosis of the patient. One size fits all.

One might reasonably ask: How does anyone know that thirty days is the right number of days to treat addiction? Is there any evidence to suggest that this number somehow represents the best way to achieve lasting sobriety? In fact there isn't. Thirty days is just a round figure borrowed from our lunar cycle—one month. As I once wrote on my blog for *Psychology Today*, "The real question is: why would people design, and defend, a treatment based on the time it takes for the moon to revolve around the earth?"[8]

And yet if we dig deeper, a second reason emerges for the thirty-day rehab. Years ago, when insurance companies used to pay for inpatient rehabilitation, it was often deemed necessary for patients to stay for much longer periods of time. Once insurance carriers set the maximum on the number of days they would cover at thirty, that quickly became the proper number of days to treat alcoholism.

Another key attribute of the rehab experience is total control. Most centers have very strict policies regarding the use of banned substances and activities. Cell phones are typically prohibited, and schedules are tightly managed. The upshot is that these thirty days represent a period of time during which patients have no choice but to stop using alcohol or other drugs. The appeal of this rule cannot be overstated: the notion of being made to stop can be a relief for both addicts and their families. Of course, living without alcohol or other drugs does not eliminate the compulsion to use them in the future. Sadly, the relief many addicts experience during hospitalization is often mirrored proportionally by the despair that follows a return to using alcohol or other drugs in the real world.

Some rehab centers will only admit those who have successfully withdrawn from alcohol or other drugs, but some also offer in-house detoxification, which is the medically monitored process of helping people withdraw safely from alcohol or other drugs. This is without question a valuable service. But even for people who are infirm medically or have certain diseases, such as diabetes, that require close monitoring during withdrawal, it is rare for detox to take longer than five days. Once the detox is complete, residential treatment is elective.

Aside from the twenty-four-hour control and monitored detox facilities, it can be difficult to find features or add-ons that necessitate the residential component of rehab programs. But that hasn't stopped these programs from creatively searching for further competitive advantages. As I described above, the nation's most famous programs have devised extraordinary lists of classes, crafts, exercises, and adventures to differentiate themselves from one another, as well as from the free 12-step meetings. These are worth considering in some further detail, both for what they promise, and for what they lack.

EXTRA FEATURES

Sierra Tucson lists on its website "qigong therapy" among its favored treatment approaches, to take just one example. Its website describes qigong as an ancient form of Tai Chi, and states that its benefits include "enhanced immune system," "increased energy and vitality," "improved intuition and creativity," "heightened spirituality," and "improved cardiovascular, respiratory, circulatory, lymphatic, and digestive function." The fact that there is no scientific basis for these claims is perhaps secondary to the more basic point that none of them have anything to do with the treatment of addiction.

Sierra Tucson also offers its guests "equine therapy," noting that the process "involves establishing a relationship with a horse on the ground and then evolves into the nurturing of that relationship, which may or may not culminate in actual riding in a contained area. . . . Horses are typically non-judgmental and have no expectations or motives. Therefore, a patient can practice congruency without the perceived fear of rejection." These claims are made without any specific reference to addiction beyond the vague intimation that being near a horse will help a person break through the "stumbling blocks to recovery."

And I'll leave this description of Sierra Tucson's Reiki treatments without comment: "Reiki involves the transfer of energy from practitioner to patient and enhances the body's natural ability to heal itself through the balancing of energy."

Sierra Tucson is hardly alone in its pursuit of novel amenities. Promises Malibu matches Sierra Tucson horse for horse with its own equine therapy program, then ups the ante with "yoga, acupuncture and massage," "life coaching," and SPECT brain imaging, a medical procedure involving injecting a radioactive chemical to visualize tumors and brain damage in dementia. The American Psychiatric Association's Psychiatric Evaluation of Adults Guideline in 2006 stated that "the use of this technique for treatment planning, diagnosis, monitoring illness or predicting prognosis has not been shown." Nor is there any known connection with addiction.

The Betty Ford Center has remained somewhat more conservative, merely offering "aquatic aerobics" and "kickboxing" among its daily activities; Passages Malibu goes all in with its "Adventure Therapy" and "Ocean Therapy" programs, the latter of which it describes as an excursion on the center's own private yacht (the *Safe Passage*), "organized to demonstrate how exciting and inspiring a sober life can be."

Put all these elements of rehab together, and it's a wonder there is any time left over for actual treatment. Indeed, a typical day in rehab may be surprising. Here is the daily schedule published by the Betty Ford Center:

Time	*Inpatient Treatment*
6:00 a.m.	• Wake Up • **Med Call** • Therapeutic Duty Assignments
7:00 a.m.	• Breakfast • Nicotine Support
8:00 a.m.	• Meditation • **Morning Lecture**
9:00 a.m.	• Process Lecture with Peers • **Community Introductions**
10:00 a.m.	• Small Group
11:00 p.m.	• Break
12:00 p.m.	• **Med Call** • Lunch
1:00 p.m.	• Relapse Prevention
2:00 p.m.	• Break/Work on Assignments
3:30 p.m.	• Fitness
5:00 p.m.	• **Med Call**
5:30 p.m.	• Dinner
6:30 p.m.	• Fitness/Free Time
7:00 p.m.	• Newcomer Meeting
8:00 p.m.	• 12-Step Meeting • Medallion Ceremony • **Med Call**
9:00 p.m.	• **Free Time**

You will notice that the day is long, running a full fifteen hours from 6 a.m. to 9 p.m. How much "treatment" is in there? There is an hour-long lecture, presumably led by a staff member; another hour-long "peer" lecture, not led by a staff member; two hour-long group meetings (a "small group" and a "relapse prevention hour"); and an hour-long 12-step meeting. Out of the fifteen-hour day, then, one can distill four actual hours of Betty Ford "treatment," half of which involve lectures instead of therapy, plus an AA meeting.

What is the rest of the day filled with? Eating, fitness, "work assignments" ("circling chairs in the group room, making community announcements, setting up tables in the dining room . . ."), and free time. There is also an hour during breakfast for "nicotine support" and a newcomer meeting when people first arrive (otherwise, patients attend the 12-step meeting).

With the possible exception of one hour ("small group"), what is notably missing from this schedule is bona fide therapy. Although there are presumably individual meetings with counselors of some sort at the Betty Ford Center—the center lists a consulting medical staff that includes physicians and psychiatrists—it apparently did not deem these critical enough to their program to be included, or even to show time for, in their daily schedule. The website confirms this in their FAQ:

> *Will I get individual sessions with my counselor?*
>
> The majority of the counseling is done in a group setting. Individual sessions occur regularly with your counselor and/or various members of the interdisciplinary treatment team, *depending on your needs.* [Emphasis added].

How typical is Betty Ford? Here is the published daily schedule from Hazelden:

> *Patients experience a full day of therapy, education and fellowship.*
> The day typically starts at 7 a.m. and ends at 8:30 p.m. and may include the following activities:
>
> • Morning meditation followed by mealtime and fellowship
> • Educational lectures followed by a group meeting for processing the lecture

- Usage history
- Twelve Step groups
- Special group meetings tailored to the needs of the individual.
  Groups could include:
  - Leisure skills group
  - Anger group
  - Stress management
  - Mental health group
  - Grief group
- Rational Emotive Therapy group
- Relaxation, exercise and recreational activities
- Individual appointments as needed with physician, psychiatrist,
  psychologist or other professional from the multidisciplinary team.
- Wellness activities such as biofeedback
- Personal time for reflection including reading and individual treat-
  ment assignments

This appears to be another long day. Yet as with Betty Ford, the "full day of therapy" promised by Hazelden actually consists largely of non-therapies such as meditation, education, relaxation, exercise, recreation, "wellness" (for example, biofeedback, for which there is no evidence of effectiveness in treating addiction), and personal time for reflection.

Most of the therapies listed consist of groups that are designated to work on certain areas or skills, and not to freely explore the individual issues for each person. Two of these are groups for "leisure skills" and "stress management," which are not directly or specifically related to the treatment of addiction. The "anger," "mental health," and grief groups may be useful for certain people but seem to be topic-focused rather than individual-focused.

The Rational Emotive Therapy group deserves special mention. RET was developed in the 1950s as an effort to look at emotional life as a problem with rationality. It is intended to help people see their irrational thoughts and learn from them. While this makes some sense, most modern frameworks of human psychology have recognized that learning one has irrational thoughts rarely solves emotional problems;

indeed, many people begin therapy knowing full well that they have irrational ideas and make poor choices, yet they cannot stop.

The Hazelden program does list individual meetings yet, like Betty Ford, describes them occurring "as needed." The explicit de-emphasis on individual therapy is common among the nation's most popular rehab programs. Even those that pay lip service to the notion of "individualized" care rarely seem to mean what most people would expect from the term. For instance, Sierra Tucson's description of its own "Individualized Treatment Plans" states: "Patients are . . . provided an individualized treatment plan, which may include disease and recovery education, relapse prevention, 12-Step meetings, Equine-Assisted Therapy, Adventure Therapy, and Grief and Spirituality therapy sessions." *Individualized* in this context seems to mean choosing different programs à la carte based on the patient. But the programs themselves are not individualized: 12-step meetings are not "individualized treatment." Educational lectures are neither individualized nor treatment. Equine therapy and adventure therapy are not recognized treatments for addiction (or anything else). And spirituality sessions are neither individual nor medical or psychological treatment. Grief counseling may be individualized if it is psychologically oriented to help people with their specific difficulties in dealing with loss, but not if it is simply generic support. Relapse prevention is a laudable goal, but if it takes place in a group setting, it is less likely to explore in any depth individual emotional factors that lead to relapse.

In sharp contrast, a good psychiatric center provides frequent individual psychotherapy for every patient. This is administered by trained psychological professionals (rather than people recovering from psychiatric problems) and is unique to the specific issues of the patient. Good psychiatric hospitals also provide psychodynamic groups whose purpose is to explore the way people interact with others in a way that is designed to bring out the singular attitudes, concerns, and difficulties unique to each person. They are not formulaic groups organized around predetermined topics. Psychiatric centers also offer sophisticated psychological testing to better understand complex or covert psychological problems and to ferret out neurobiological issues such as learning or attention disorders.

How did standardized, education-like group therapy become the predominant mode of treatment at rehab centers, despite their having ample room and money to employ a higher standard of professional care? One clue might be to examine the credentials and expertise of the staff.

Many staff members at rehabilitation centers have extremely limited training. Although every program boasts of the presence of psychologists and psychiatrists in a consulting capacity, many of those who provide direct treatment are qualified mainly by being "in recovery." This is not a terribly difficult credential to attain: Hazelden's own website invites visitors to "Become an addiction counselor in as little as one year." Training to be a clinical social worker, psychologist, or psychiatrist, by contrast, requires from three to eight years, and to be an excellent therapist takes years beyond the end of formal training.

Also noteworthy is that although many rehab programs have psychiatrists or psychologists on speed dial, these people virtually never become the primary therapists for patients, instead serving in supervisory or consultative roles. To this day there are no academic requirements for becoming a counselor or "therapist" in a drug-rehabilitation facility.

A 2007 exposé in the *Los Angeles Times* noted: "Promises and fierce rival Passages Addiction Cure Center make sweeping claims on their websites about their clinical successes and reputations, purporting to have few or no equals in the world. Addiction researchers say the boasts are virtually impossible to substantiate. In addition, Promises, Passages, and other Malibu rehab firms have identified on their websites a number of psychiatrists and other physicians as staff members, even though the centers are not licensed to provide medical care."[9]

The issue here goes deeper than the value of good training. There is considerable evidence to support the idea that counselors without professional backgrounds develop their own personal ideas about what constitutes appropriate treatment and philosophy. For example, nonprofessionally trained "recovering" addicts in AA, who often provide treatment for addiction in this country, tend to tell patients to do what they themselves did, since they have neither training nor experience with anything else.

Untrained counselors may do more harm than good. One study surveyed 317 staff members of hospital-based residential detoxification and rehabilitation programs, nonhospital detoxification and rehabilitation centers, outpatient and intensive outpatient drug-free clinics, methadone maintenance clinics, freestanding recovery houses, and several specialized inpatient and outpatient programs for adolescents, women, and women with children.[10] The authors found that "[i]ndividuals with more formal training tended to be less supportive of confrontation. . . . Support for the increased use of confrontation was strongest among staff members with the least formal education." The significance of this is that confrontation is basically a nonprofessional stance, in contrast with understanding, or often even trying to understand, what drives people to behaviors they themselves wish they could stop. Too often, it is also an enactment of these untrained counselors' frustration with patients. The authors appropriately deplored this finding, writing, "Perhaps staff rely upon confrontational approaches because they are unfamiliar with alternatives . . . beliefs about the utility of confrontation may be subject to change based on education . . . senior clinicians might be most easily enlisted to implement, and possibly help transfer, these less confrontational approaches."

Another recent paper examined 592 treatment providers in the United States and United Kingdom and found that the belief that addiction is a disease was stronger among those who provide for-profit treatment, have stronger spiritual beliefs, and have had a past addiction problem.[11] One would hope that what treaters believe about addiction would arise not from these factors but from knowledge—just the thing professional training provides.

MONEY AND EFFECTIVENESS

Of course, there is one more difference between rehab and traditional 12-step programs: money. Most rehabilitation centers are extraordinary financial enterprises, charging more in a few months than the most expensive universities charge for a full year of tuition. Even those that are legally nonprofits seem somehow to justify large monthly rates. Hazelden charges around $28,300 a month and notes that "additional services such as counseling for other issues, prescriptions, etc. are charged separately when needed." The Betty Ford Center charges $32,000 for thirty days, not counting detoxification. Sierra Tucson starts its residential program at $39,000 for thirty days, but the price leaps to $2,300 a day ($69,000 a month) for residents in the "Medical Assessment and Stabilization Unit." Promises Malibu's prices range from $55,000 for a shared room and up to $90,000 a month for a private suite. Passages Malibu starts at $88,500 for a twenty-eight-day stay.

One of the principal ways that these facilities justify their price tags is with outsized claims of effectiveness. Yet, the industry regularly does not provide this data. I made a direct inquiry to Dr. A. Thomas McClellan, the chief executive officer of the Treatment Research Center that has for years done research for Betty Ford. He replied: "We have done work for them for quite a while but there is to my knowledge no follow up study—at least in the past ten years." The response to the same inquiry put to a different rehab, Sierra Tucson, was that they had no outcome data at all. As one addiction researcher put it in the *Los Angeles Times*, "Anybody can make any claim they want and get away with it. It's essentially an unregulated industry."[12] McClellan told the *New York Times*, "It doesn't really matter if you're a movie star going to some resort by the sea or a homeless person. The system doesn't work well for what for many people is a chronic, recurring problem." The *New York Times* put it this way in 2008:

> Very few rehabilitation programs have the evidence to show that they are effective. The resort-and-spa private clinics generally do not allow outside researchers to verify their published success rates. The publicly supported programs spend their scarce resources on patient care, not costly studies.
>
> And the field has no standard guidelines. Each program has its own philosophy; so, for that matter, do individual counselors. No one knows which approach is best for which patient, because these

programs rarely if ever track clients closely after they graduate. Even Alcoholics Anonymous, the best known of all the substance-abuse programs, does not publish data on its participants' success rate.[13]

Rehab programs thrive in this gray area.

THE DATA

Hazelden is a slight exception, having been far more forthcoming than many other rehab programs in describing and studying its own outcomes. On its website, Hazelden has reported that at one month following discharge, over 20 percent of patients said that they had resumed drinking; at six months, that number had risen to over 40 percent; and at one year, almost 50 percent of patients had resumed drinking.[14] Although there is no data beyond one year, the downward slope of this outcome suggests that fewer than half of these former inpatients remained abstinent after the first year. This is a troubling result. But as it turns out, even these findings have been inflated.

Hazelden's abstinence figures are taken from a 1998 article published in the *Journal of Addictive Behaviors*.[15] The study involved people who had gone through the Hazelden rehab and then followed up at one, six, and twelve months. None of these patients were interviewed in person; instead, all were sent questionnaires by mail. If patients did not return the questionnaire, they were called on the telephone. All of the data was therefore captured from self-report or the reports of people whom patients had chosen to reply for them.

The limitations of this method are obvious: people who are not doing well often will not reveal the extent of their return to addictive behavior because of shame, an unwillingness to acknowledge that they have not succeeded in the caller's program, or hostility to telling the truth to somebody they don't know. Consequently, it is far easier to get false positive results from this sort of study design (people claiming to be doing better than they are) than false negatives (people claiming to be doing worse than they are). But even more problematic than the tendency of self-reports to underreport bad results is what the researchers did with those who failed to respond at all. Unlike Hazelden's summary, the paper itself reveals that the authors ignored the critically large attrition rate in their subjects. They reported the results of only the people they could contact, and did not count those who dropped out. It is well known in survey-based research that those who drop out tend to be those who fared worst; indeed, the paper's authors made this very point, even though they fell into this error:

> Outcome figures may be considered to represent the upper limits of outcome . . . the self-administered mailed questionnaires were completed and returned by those individuals who could easily be contacted and who were willing to complete the questionnaire. If someone did not respond to the mailing, then the telephone follow-up method was initiated. These individuals may not have responded to the mailing because they did not want to report that they had used alcohol during the follow-up period. These results are corroborated by other studies showing that easy-to-contact subjects have better outcomes than do difficult-to-contact subjects. Therefore, those clients who were not contacted with either follow-up method are more likely to have poorer outcomes, as a group than those who were contacted.[16]

How many people were unaccounted for? The authors again: "The outcome figures are based on 1-month, 6-month, and 1-year follow-up response rates of 79%, 76%, and 71% of the sample, respectively. . . . About one-quarter of the sample remains unaccounted for in terms of follow-up outcome data." The authors also found that the people who didn't return the mailed questionnaire and had to be contacted by phone showed poorer outcomes than those who did return the questionnaire, giving further support to the notion that the people most eager to respond were those with the best outcomes.

What happens to the data if everyone is included? We cannot know whether all the dropouts resumed drinking, but as all researchers (including the authors) agree, it is likely that they did worse as a group. Let's start by assuming that all the dropouts resumed drinking. Then, using the reported percent of dropouts at each measuring point, here are the results with everyone counted: *At one month, nearly 40 percent of patients resumed drinking. At six months, about 55 percent resumed drinking. At one year, 63 percent of patients had resumed drinking.*

These results paint an even grimmer picture than Hazelden's presentation of the data. But, just as Hazelden's numbers overestimate its success, these numbers may overstate its failure. So let's recalculate with an optimistic assumption in Hazelden's favor. Let us assume that, instead of all of the dropouts resuming drinking, they had only mildly worse outcomes, say 25 percent worse than the measured group. Then the numbers look like this: *At one month, about 27 percent of patients had resumed drinking. At six months, the number rises to about 44 percent. By one year, 51 percent resumed drinking.*

The correct numbers are probably somewhere between these two results. But even with this more optimistic reading of the data, one year after a rehabilitation treatment whose stated aim is the AA goal of abstinence, most patients had returned to drinking. Given the downward direction of the data, we can reasonably conclude that if the study were continued beyond one year, the outcome would continue to worsen. For a lifetime problem, this is a serious deficiency.

Hazelden opted to present its data another way as well, reporting findings about the percentage of days abstinent (PDA), rather than complete abstinence. This actually makes a good deal of sense from a treatment perspective, since patients can improve without being continuously abstinent. Looking at days without drinking, Hazelden's ex-patients reported significant improvement at all the follow-ups within the first year, although as with continuous abstinence, the improvement declined over time. Hazelden shows a graph of these apparently excellent results on its website, though the reference for this graph is not given. Without seeing the data behind the graph, we cannot know what the PDA data mean in real terms. But we know that the numbers Hazelden used for its presentation are averages; they don't include breakdowns of how many patients were drinking large amounts, how many were drinking medium amounts, and how many patients were abstinent. And given the way data was gathered and treated in the *Journal of Addictive Behaviors* paper just cited, we cannot know whether these are all self-reports by questionnaire or whether the dropouts in the study were counted.

However, we can look at the same PDA data from the *Journal of Addictive Behaviors* paper just examined, since PDA results were also described there. That paper found that at one year 16 percent of the non-dropout patients drank at least one day weekly. Once again, however, the authors do not account for the 420 of the original 1,083 people who dropped out of this portion of the study. If we again assume they did less well than the people who responded and drank at least one day weekly, the percentage of patients who were weekly drinkers after one year more than triples—to 49 percent. If we recalculate with the same optimistic view of the dropout group that we used before (that the dropouts' weekly drinking was only 25 percent more than the measured group), the weekly drinking figure rises to over 18 percent. Somewhere between 18 percent and 49 percent represents a dismaying proportion of people who were drinking every week twelve months after leaving rehab. And this number, of course, is derived from data biased toward favorable self-reports. Finally, this result doesn't include all those (the majority, as we saw above) who are drinking, even if not every single week.

What can we conclude from this? At minimum, as the researchers themselves write (with some understatement), "There appears to be a loss of treatment effect over time." It appears that the benefits of being away from the stresses of ordinary life, in a beautiful and peaceful setting with caring people, exercise, good food, lectures, and topic-focused discussion groups, do not last long. And besides these generic supports, the single foundational treatment offered by Hazelden and most other rehab centers is the 12-step program, whose success rate we know. Rehab's poor outcomes in light of these limitations are, therefore, not surprising.

Besides the Hazelden studies, there is little academic literature on rehab treatment outcomes. One paper cited in chapter 3 does apply, though: the 2003 study by McKellar and colleagues. In that investigation, you will recall, the subjects (all men) had been treated in a 12-step *inpatient* program before being followed up. After one year, "hazardous consumption" (the frequency of consuming more than four drinks on a drinking day) was still extremely high, at 42 percent. Even this very troubling result is certain to be an underestimate: this study suffered from the same major positive biases as the Hazelden paper, relying on self-reports and excluding those (nearly 25 percent) who had dropped out. An accurate estimate of hazardous drinking was probably at or above 50 percent at one year, consistent with the corrected Hazelden data.

It cannot be ignored that the nation's best-known rehabs seem to continually fail their highest-profile clients as well, as most Americans with a passing familiarity with popular culture will know. Boldfaced names such as Charlie Sheen, Lindsay Lohan, Robert Downey Jr., Britney Spears, and the late Whitney Houston have, according to the media, been through rehab many times. Amy Winehouse famously wrote a song rejecting a return to rehab just a few years before she died of substance abuse. Danny Bonaduce once said about Promises Malibu: "They charged me more than $40,000 for my stay and I drank on the way home. But Malibu was beautiful. I remember thinking that if this place had a bar, it would be fantastic."[17] With the 2013 death of Mindy McCready, the number of deaths associated with the hit show *Celebrity Rehab* reached five, leading Dr. Drew Pinsky to shutter the operation.

CONSEQUENCES OF FAILURE

There is a certain halo around the rehab industry that can make its failures all the more poignant. Because many people can't buy into AA for various reasons, including its religiosity, its rigidity, and its close-mindedness to criticism or different ideas, rehabs centered on the Twelve Steps may produce significant conflict within people as they struggle to get help. The mandatory requirement to attend 12-step meetings and the pressure to accept AA philosophy in the great majority of rehab centers have likely led many a patient to feel unheard. And when they relapse after leaving expensive and triumphantly marketed programs, the experience can lead to hopelessness. The Betty Ford Center writes on its website, "Alcoholics, addicts, and their loved ones who require alcohol treatment or drug treatment begin the exciting journey to a new life at the Betty Ford Center." Sierra Tucson's site says that at their "internationally-renowned alcohol treatment center, you won't just be undergoing alcohol rehab. During your time at Sierra Tucson, you will experience innovative alcohol treatment programs that can effectively treat you completely." Promises Malibu's site states, "Promises drug rehab centers create the ultimate safe-haven for you or your loved one who has decided to take this important step: choosing to create an extraordinary life." We can only imagine the pain of seeing the dream of a new life dissolve into the difficult patterns of the old.

The overwrought marketing literature of most rehab programs is intentionally designed to sell a fantasy, placing them in marked contrast to organizations whose descriptions are guided by professional standards of honesty and decorum. No respected hospital or program would claim to be able to so transform the people who enter its doors. And all of them acknowledge that if a patient isn't better upon completion of the treatment, it's not the patient's fault.

For instance, here is the self-description of one of the nation's finest medical facilities: "The mission of Dana-Farber Cancer Institute is to provide expert, compassionate care to children and adults with cancer while advancing the understanding, diagnosis, treatment, cure, and prevention of cancer and related diseases." And here's one of the country's finest psychiatric facilities: "For over 90 years, the Austen Riggs Center has offered long-term residential and hospital-level psychiatric treatment based on intensive, four-times-weekly individual psychotherapy, provided by psychiatrists and psychologists who have advanced and specialized training."[18]

The consequences of a post-rehab relapse are often far greater because of the enormous costs, as well. For many families who are making a major financial sacrifice based partly on the promise of metamorphic treatment, seeing a loved one return to addiction can be devastating. Patients have too often found that their support networks are not as robust following a stint at rehab; it's not uncommon for families to direct their resentment when a patient "fails" not toward the rehab, but toward the patient: "How could he return to drinking after we put him through that wonderful/famous program at such expense?" And let us remind ourselves that this expense is usually borne without insurance.

THE AMERICAN SANITARIUM LIVES ON

In a sense, rehab centers are hardly new. They occupy a specific place in the American imagination that has thrived for more than a century: the mythology of the convalescent paradise.

Chronic diseases requiring chronic care have been with us throughout history. To take just one example, one hundred years ago, a pandemic of tuberculosis led to the rise of TB sanitaria. Often these were placed in warm, dry climates with "clean air" where breathing was easier. A close look at these lovely facilities provides a number of startling parallels to the addiction rehab industry that would follow a century later. Because TB was so widespread, many of its sufferers had enough money to choose any inpatient center they wished. This created a competitive market, and TB sanitaria marketed themselves with ever more elaborate treatment programs offering high-end luxuries sought by those who could afford them. A look at some of the marketing literature of the day feels eerily familiar:

Here is the Battle Creek Sanitarium, in 1907: "The one institution where all the most recent scientific curative measures have been assembled under one control. Many new and interesting departments have been recently installed, including Radium, Diathermy, Electrical Exercises . . . the Sanitarium offers many unique opportunities to health-seekers. The new Diet System, the physical culture classes . . . the interesting health lectures, swimming, games and drills."[19]

The Sanitarium at Dansville, New York, enticed visitors with its "Beautiful Location among the hills of Genesee Valley. Pure air, pure water; climate especially mild and equable at all seasons of the year. . . . It has light, airy rooms. . . . All forms of baths, electricity, massage, etc. are scientifically administered. The apparatus for Dr. Taylor's Swedish Movements, and a superior Holtz machine for Statical Electricity are special features. . . . An unrivalled Health Resort."[20]

And so on. Moore's Brook Sanitarium called itself a "splendid old Colonial place, over 100 acres, mature grove, grass and vine . . . 250 feet of wide veranda . . . Billiards, pool, golf, tennis, etc." And Dr. Rogers' Hydropathic Sanitarium and Congenial Home noted its "fine grounds and salubrious air" that could "effectually remove any disease, however chronic."[21]

Despite these luxuries, none of these institutions offered any treatment for the actual cause of the illness. Indeed, while the bacterium causing TB was discovered in 1882, it would be sixty-four years before any real treatment (an effective antibiotic) was developed. It was precisely during these years when the TB sanitaria thrived. Once specific treatment did become available, the elaborate sanitaria died out, never to return.

Alcohol and drug rehabilitation centers are in just this position now, with one marked difference. Better understanding and treatment are already available; they are just not included in their programs. The addiction treatment industry is based on a model that has been unchanged since the 1930s, and because these programs are commonly staffed by people who often know little beyond AA and whose professional identities depend on the rightness of that model, there has been an enormous resistance to change. This failure in understanding and treating addiction is plainly evident in the proliferation of strange therapies and unrecognized treatments, which rehabs continue to hawk.

What might a better rehab program look like? To begin with, instead of the senseless notion of requiring exactly the same number of days of hospitalization for everyone, a rational program would be individualized. Considering that one purpose of residential care is to provide a more intensive treatment, all patients would be seen by an experienced, well-trained psychotherapist multiple times a week, if not daily. Therapists would have to be professionally qualified academically and up to standards of excellence for psychotherapists in the community.

Groups would be a highly valuable component, if they were designed to help patients learn about themselves and how they relate to others; that is, to find out how they are perceived and to experiment with new ways of relating. Patients themselves would bring up the ways their addiction has intertwined with their feelings about themselves and their relationships with others; no meeting would come with a set "educational" agenda.

An ideal program would also have no need for lectures about drugs or for instruction about how to use 12-step programs. Alcoholics Anonymous would be made available outside the center (free of charge, of course) for those who could make good use of it. Any decent program would also provide basic services such as adequate food and common spaces for patients to talk and learn from each other. But gourmet food and spectacular settings have nothing to do with treating addiction, so these frills would be eliminated, allowing the cost of rehabilitation to stay within reach of the common person.

I will say more about effective treatment, after first considering what really does make sense in understanding and treating addiction, in the next chapter.

CHAPTER FIVE

SO, WHAT *DOES* WORK TO TREAT ADDICTION?

BECAUSE THE NATURE OF *addiction* itself has never really been understood in human history, the phenomenon was originally associated only with its clearest form: drunkenness. The symptoms of inebriation were easy to see, leading to the conclusion that alcoholism was about the physical effects of alcohol. Because alcoholics not only couldn't stop, but often enjoyed their drinking despite its terrible effects on others and themselves, many people also believed that alcoholism was a moral failing, even a kind of insanity. These ideas—that the problem of alcoholism lay in the power of alcohol, and that alcoholics had a moral deficit that allowed them to succumb to this power—led to a treatment that pressed alcoholics to acknowledge the power of this chemical and try to improve their morality by turning to God. This approach was, of course, Alcoholics Anonymous.

One of the principal sources of confusion was that people mixed up *physical addiction* with the underlying *nature* of addiction. Even though both may be present in the same person at the same time, they actually have nothing to do with each other. Physical addiction is a simple physiological phenomenon that can happen to anybody. Our bodies react to certain drugs by adapting to them, changing to accommodate their presence. This phenomenon is called *tolerance*. Dramatic things can happen when people stop taking a drug to which they have become tolerant. Because the body is "prepared" to deal with the drug, when the drug is removed, a reaction occurs. The body pushes back, compensating for a drug that isn't there.

This is known as a *withdrawal syndrome*—a set of physiological symptoms that are always expressed in the exact opposite direction from the effects of the drug. Since nearly every drug capable of producing physical addiction is a sedative (also known as a central nervous system depressant, or "downer"), the withdrawal syndrome is physiological overexcitement. In the case of alcohol, this starts with shaking ("the shakes"), but can proceed to full-blown seizures. Withdrawal from other drugs looks different. Narcotic withdrawal, for instance, commonly involves goose bumps and severe gastrointestinal discomfort. Interestingly, since seizures aren't present for narcotic withdrawal, it's actually medically safer to withdraw from heroin than from alcohol.

How do we know that this physical addiction has nothing to do with the true nature of addiction? One clue is that many addictions have no physical component at all. Examples include the addictive use of marijuana or LSD, which don't produce a tolerance response, and all the non-drug addictions such as compulsive gambling, eating, shopping, and sex. A second clue is that it's common to develop a *physical addiction* but never have a true addiction. Everyone who is hospitalized and given high enough doses of morphine over a period of enough time to treat pain—for example as part of treatment for cancer—will become physically addicted. But when these people are discharged, they generally don't run out and find the local drug pusher. One more way to be sure that physical addiction and true addiction are separate things: we know from vast experience that, even after detoxification, when there is no more physical addiction, true addicts are not "cured" of their need to use alcohol or other drugs. Many return to use months or even years after detox.

THE BEGINNING OF MODERN UNDERSTANDING

Starting in the 1960s, experts in human psychology began to take an interest in addiction for the first time. Rather than viewing the behavior as a form of pleasure seeking, they theorized that taking drugs was something people did to manage intolerable feelings, almost like self-prescribing a medication. Thus was born the now-famous "self-medication hypothesis" of drug use.

Over time, other ideas about the psychology of addiction were developed, expanding and improving on this early insight. In the decades of my practice with patients with addictions, I noted that addiction as a behavior was very much like another common psychological symptom: *compulsions*, a category that includes other common unwished-for acts like having to arrange papers parallel to each other on a desk or having to excessively clean house. Many of these compulsions aren't nearly as dangerous or destructive as addictions, of course; maddening as they might be, they are unlikely to result in a car accident or drunken brawl or do damage to vital organs. But even though the consequences may be less severe, these compulsive behaviors might share psychological roots with addictions. After all, by definition, compulsions are driven behaviors that people cannot stop themselves from doing, even when they want to. And so the question arose: what if addiction is just the name we give to compulsions that involve drugs?

(A word of clarification is needed here. There are compulsive behaviors that are not primarily psychological in origin: those described by the diagnosis *obsessive-compulsive disorder*, or OCD. The compulsions produced in OCD typically respond to medications such as Prozac and its SSRI cousins. In contrast, *psychologically based* compulsive behaviors do not respond to the Prozac group, since they have a psychological cause. Unlike the OCD symptoms, these compulsions are triggered by emotional factors and can be treated in psychotherapy. Depression is another example of a symptom that can have two separate causes. There is biochemical depression, which is caused by low levels of neurotransmitters and treatable by medication. And there is psychological depression, which does not respond to antidepressants but is treatable by psychotherapy.)

The idea that drug addictions (including alcoholism) are just compulsions focused on drugs had good support. In the early 1970s, researcher Lee Robins and her group looked at heroin addiction in soldiers who had returned from Vietnam.[1] Many soldiers had used heroin extensively and in high doses during the war. In fact, the abuse was so widespread that when they returned to the States, soldiers were routinely screened for heroin addiction. Those who had a physical addiction to the drug were detoxified before returning to their homes.

At the same time soldiers were using so much heroin overseas, there was an explosion of heroin use in the United States (this is when the term "hooked on drugs" first arose). Yet there was a fascinating difference between these two cohorts of drug users. The stateside addicts had virtually no success maintaining abstinence after they were done with detox, which was what had led to the widespread fear that the nation was becoming irrevocably "hooked." But Robins found, to the surprise of many, that just six months after coming home, over 90 percent of the veterans had quit using heroin. This seemed like an impossible result. After all, if heroin was so addictive, how could its fabled power fade immediately for some people and linger for others?

A logical question arose: were the stateside heroin addicts and the soldiers using the same drug? It turned out that, if anything, there was evidence that the heroin available in Vietnam was actually *more* powerful than its stateside counterpart. So there had to be something about the *people* that was different.

What was this difference? The soldiers used heroin because they were at war, with all its unthinkable horrors. Heroin helped them to deal with this external reality; once that reality evaporated, they no longer needed the drug. But the stateside addicts used heroin for completely different reasons—because it served an emotional purpose for them, just like any other compulsive behavior. Their war was in a sense internal; their drug use was driven by enduring psychological issues, not temporary circumstantial ones. These were the true addicts, the ones who couldn't quit.

The Robins study became a landmark in the recognition of the idea that compulsive drug use has nothing fundamentally to do with the *physical action* of the drug; it has to do with the *psychology* of its use. This was clear evidence that addiction was more about something in people's minds, not something in the chemicals they used. Thinking about this now, it seems obvious—as I said, large numbers of people develop physical dependencies on prescribed drugs every year and do not go on to become addicts once the prescription runs out.

In case further evidence was warranted, another massive natural experiment around the same time drove the point home. In 1970, the surgeon general mandated that all cigarette packs carry a warning label about the dangers of smoking; in 1985, this label was hardened with specific mentions of lung cancer, heart disease, and emphysema. When these warnings appeared, millions of people stopped smoking, even though they had been physically addicted to the nicotine in cigarettes.[2] Just like the soldiers in Vietnam, many had been smoking for reasons other than a psychological compulsion—enjoyment, for one—which meant they could relatively easily decide to stop when they realized it was dangerous for them to smoke.

Once again, even for a drug known to cause physical addiction like heroin or nicotine, taking it in very high quantities for a long time could not cause people to become addicts if they also didn't have a psychological need to use the drug.

By the mid-1980s, the self-medication concept had become largely solidified among clinicians and researchers studying addiction.[3] And soon a new piece of evidence began to gain recognition: people often switched between drug addictions and non-drug addictions. As many as 75 percent of compulsive gamblers have some alcohol abuse history, for example.[4] Many people switch between the addictive use of drugs and non-chemical addictions such as Internet use and shopping. This would be inexplicable if addiction were about drugs or their effects. Yet it makes perfect sense when addiction is viewed through the prism of *function*: it is clearly doing something for these people emotionally. And in this sense, almost any behavior will do.

RISE OF THE BIOLOGISTS

But just as a consensus was beginning to develop around the psychology of addiction, a new hypothesis entered the fray. A group of scientists at the National Institute on Drug Abuse (NIDA) began to publish a series of studies in the first decade of this century devoted to the *neurobiology* of addiction. They eventually declared that they had discovered the biological basis of addiction.

The NIDA scientists have been tremendously successful from a public relations standpoint. Journalists who rely on big announcements to drive interest have repeated the NIDA's bold claims ad nauseam, and as a result many lay people now believe the idea that addiction is an issue of brain chemistry. The power of this idea is its aura of rigor. Neurobiology is often described as *hard science*—the researchers use the very latest imaging tools and technologies, and their literature comes complete with numbers and beautiful images of the brain "lighting up." Compared with the "soft science" of psychology, these stories feel far more modern and accurate. But are they?

Here is what the researchers found. They began by addicting rats to heroin. Then they showed those rats "cues" that had been present at the time they received heroin and were therefore associated with the drug—a play on Pavlov, with heroin instead of biscuits. Soon these cues excited the rats even when the drug wasn't present, confirming that the researchers had successfully created a "conditioned reflex." Then the NIDA researchers did something new: they examined the rats' brains. And what they discovered was that these brains had actually changed as a result of exposure to the drug. Specifically, their brains secreted more of a neurotransmitter called dopamine in response to the cues, which triggered the "reward" or "pleasure" pathway of the brain. They then noted something else: this brain change, called *upregulation*, since it involved an excessive response to a stimulus, was permanent. Once the rats' brains had become upregulated, they would never return to normal. The researchers concluded from this evidence that addiction must therefore be a "chronic brain disease" caused by taking significant amounts of a drug. And even though these tests did not involve people, the researchers announced that they had discovered the cause of addiction in humans.[5]

This conclusion was problematic in several ways, but the biggest by far was that it fits virtually nothing we know about human addiction. For example, recall the Vietnam veterans study once again. Those soldiers had taken significant quantities of heroin over a long period of time, far more than enough to create a physical addiction to the drug. If we subscribed to the "chronic brain disease" theory, then those soldiers should have undergone a permanent brain change that rendered them addicts forever. In fact, only a small percentage of these users became addicted at any time after their return.[6] The same thing happened when those warning labels appeared on cigarette packs: millions quit, despite the fact that their usage patterns should have upregulated them into a lifetime of subservience to tobacco. People stopped smoking because they realized that smoking is dangerous, and because they *could* stop. None of this fits the profile of a chronic brain disease.

And we have an even larger sample to disprove the neurobiological model: alcoholism itself. Close to 100 percent of adults in America drink alcohol. Many people drink in large quantities for many years, especially when they're younger. Many such people drink enough to become physically dependent. Yet despite enormous exposure over many years, the vast majority of younger heavy drinkers never become alcoholics. If the "chronic brain disease" theory were correct, they all would be.

And consider once more the millions of people whose prescription drug use for temporary or chronic pain produces powerful tolerance and withdrawal. The vast majority of these people do not go on to become addicts; the chronic brain disease theory should see them upregulated into a life of permanent addiction.

What happened is that the NIDA researchers made a critical, and critically false, assumption. Knowing that all mammals share essentially the same reward system in the brain, they assumed that humans exposed to drugs in high doses over long periods would develop the same response: given heavy enough exposure, people would run around helplessly seeking the drug like rats in a cage. But what they overlooked was precisely what makes humans different from rats. On top of our pleasure pathway, we have a very large "higher" brain. We humans almost always do things not just because we are physically excited by them, but because of a very complex mechanism we possess that rats do not. This mechanism is psychology.

As evidence, consider that unlike rats, humans often become calmer at the moment they *decide* to have a drink, or *choose* to call their dealer, or *plan* a trip to the casino. Tranquil hours may pass between decision and delivery. The fact that the mere act of deciding seems to calm our nerves suggests that this act has some psychological significance to us. (More on this in a moment.)

There is another essential fact about human addiction that has gone ignored by the NIDA team: humans regularly perform addictive acts in response to being emotionally upset. A broken relationship, a stinging defeat, a painful incident that causes guilt or shame—these are common precipitants of addictive acts in humans. We are complex creatures who are governed as much by our thoughts and feelings as by our reptilian pleasure pathways. To reduce human addiction to the physiological excitement of rats is to dismiss everything that makes us human.

Finally, what the rat researchers call *automatic behavior*—running around seeking heroin upon exposure to cues in their environment— is a conditioned reflex with a neurobiological basis, similar to *seeking behavior*—when people are in physical withdrawal and need to get to their drug. But this automatic behavior has simply nothing to do with addiction, and should never have been called *addiction* to begin with.

THE GENETICISTS

Closely related to the neurobiologists are the geneticists, who are often the sources for mass media reports announcing the good news that we have finally found the gene for alcoholism. (People seem to find this gene so often that one wonders how they manage to keep losing it.) Confusion has arisen because of some findings that suggest that for *some* people with alcoholism, there is some genetic "loading"; that is, a degree to which the diagnosis correlates with genetic inheritance. But this should not be taken as evidence that there is a gene for alcoholism or addiction or that addiction is somehow a genetic disorder.

The problem comes down to confusion between causation and correlation once again. Statistically, it is likely that many genes, possibly hundreds or thousands of them, may play some role in increasing the *susceptibility* to addiction. This has led some researchers to refer to *susceptibility genes*. But nobody has ever discovered any of these genes, despite the fact that they have been repeatedly sleuthed by our most sophisticated chromosomal techniques. I reviewed the best-known genetic studies in my book *The Heart of Addiction*, but I'd like to repeat just one salient point here.[7]

One of the most popular tools in genetics is the identical-twin study—popular because it allows researchers to study two different people with exactly the same genes. Twin studies have revealed that if one twin has alcoholism, it is more likely than not (greater than 50 percent chance) that the other twin does *not* have alcoholism. This would be an impossible finding in the case of a true genetic disease, of course. It's true that evidence shows that if one twin is an alcoholic, the other has about a 40 percent chance of having alcoholism too, which is higher than the general population.[8] But when we consider that the identical twins in these studies were raised simultaneously by the same parents, at the same time, in the same environment, and typically have very similar experiences growing up, the increased correlation (called *concordance* in genetic studies) is to be expected.

In fact, there is probably some genetic influence on addictions, but this shouldn't be surprising. Many human conditions, like peptic ulcer disease or hypertension, have some genetic loading, meaning that genes confer some degree of increased susceptibility without the condition being directly heritable. Given the way addiction works psychologically, it could be possible that some decreased biological tolerance of certain emotions could lead to a variety of symptoms, including addiction. But nobody in human history has ever walked into a bar because a gene told them to.

THE PSYCHOLOGY OF ADDICTION

Now let us return to the compulsion model. The idea fits neatly with much that has been written about addiction for centuries. People have understood the basic nature of compulsions for a long time, even before modern psychology. William Shakespeare provided an especially clear example in *Macbeth*: Lady Macbeth demonstrates literature's most quotable compulsion when she wails "Out, damned spot!" while ceaselessly washing her hands. The "spot" that she imagines is the blood of people she has murdered, of course, and her compulsive behavior is universally comprehensible in human terms: a symbolic gesture to undo her guilt. Because she can't actually reverse the murders, the compulsion becomes a stand-in for the act itself: cleanse the hands if you can't raise the dead. In psychology, there is a word for an action like this that substitutes for a more direct behavior: a *displacement*.

It is understood in psychology that all compulsions are displacements. One of their defining features is how irrational they seem; in the inner world of our minds, the direct act and its substitute may be adequate surrogates, but to everyone else they can seem crazy. Yet compulsions can be relieved by undoing the displacement. If a real Lady Macbeth had dealt with her guilt more directly (that is, by confessing to the victims' relatives, or asking for forgiveness, or even just coming to some peace by thinking through her behavior), then she might have been liberated from the need to endlessly repeat her handwashing.

Once addictive behavior is defined through the prism of compulsive behavior,[9] it can be treated just as psychotherapists would treat any emotionally driven compulsion, using talk therapy to root out the deeper meanings and purposes behind the behavior.[10] (Again, I am making a distinction between chemical OCD and psychological compulsions, which are wholly different in their origin and treatment.) There is no longer any reason to appeal to a Higher Power, to think of addiction as its own "disease," or to rely solely on fellow addicts for relief. No one would ever treat a housecleaning compulsion by relying on the been-there-done-that counsel of recovering housecleaners or suggest that compulsive housecleaning is a spiritual problem.

MARION'S CASE

The easiest way to explain the psychology of addictions, as I have uncovered it over the past twenty-five years, is to show it. The following vignette is a short version of a case story that originally appeared in my book *The Heart of Addiction*.[11]

Marion put down the phone after hearing her husband's command to prepare dinner for him and a group of business guests that evening. She had always hated these dinners, but as usual, she had responded to his request by saying "Yes, of course." Now she would have to shop and hurry around prepping the house. As she stood there, she felt the familiar, nearly overwhelming, urge to take some of her Percodans. She walked over to the medicine cabinet, took out her pills and swallowed two of them.

For personal reasons that echoed from her past, Marion felt unable to defy her husband's insistent demands. But this inability to speak up left her with a terrible feeling—an agonizing sensation, like being caught in a trap. She would have liked nothing better than to tell Gerry to make his own damn dinner. But she felt she just couldn't. Like anybody faced with a sense of overwhelming helplessness, she had to do *something* to get out of the trap. And for her, that something had always been taking her pills.

This is what addiction is about.

When Marion took her pills, she felt better. Yes, the medication had a soothing effect, but that wasn't the whole story. She noticed that she started to feel better long before the drug could possibly have an effect; Marion felt better even before she took the pills. Indeed, like every addict I have ever met, Marion started to feel better at the moment she *decided* to take the drug. How could this be possible?

The answer is deceptively simple: she had already solved her problem. Of course, she hadn't done anything about the dinner or about Gerry. But she had solved her internal problem—the sense of intolerable helplessness. By deciding to take a pill, Marion had chosen to do something within her own control, something that would make her feel better. Gone was the unbearable sense of powerlessness, replaced by a liberating sense of control. This phenomenon repeats across all addictions. And this fact helps us to see the first piece of the addiction puzzle: *The psychological function of addiction is to reverse the sense of overwhelming helplessness.*

This may sound counterintuitive at first. After all, we know that addiction regularly leads people to experience more, not less, helplessness in their lives. But that's because of the awful consequences of addiction, and consequences have little to do with the act in the moment. The drive to reverse utter helplessness is an explosive force, the natural human rage to fight against being trapped. We know this kind of anger has the capacity to overwhelm a person's judgment while she is in the throes of it. Emotions this strong have compelled many people to do things they later regretted terribly.

I often use the example of people caught in a cave-in to illustrate the experience of utter helplessness that precipitates addictive acts. When two hundred tons of rock suddenly fall between you and daylight, you might try to stay calm. But it won't last forever. The time will come when you begin pounding at the rocks, clawing at the boulders and hurling yourself against the walls with enough abandon that you might even break a few bones. This is *normal*, an understandable reaction with evolutionary survival value. Nobody would accuse you of being self-destructive for breaking your wrist in an intense effort to get out of the cave.[12] And this rage at helplessness boils up equally when people feel emotionally trapped, like Marion. It is what gives addiction its most defining characteristic: an enormous intensity that overrides every other concern and good judgment, and that often seems impossible to stop by either the person herself or those around her. And so this delivers the second piece of the puzzle: *If reversal of helplessness is the* function *of addiction, then the powerful* drive *behind addiction is rage at that helplessness.*

But there is one remaining question in Marion's story. We know the function of her addiction and the drive behind it, but why pills? Why do people do things that have no realistic chance of solving the problem? Pills are just one example; others have a drink or go out looking for sex. And this brings us back to where we started: with the idea of displacement. Marion couldn't take the direct step of standing up to Gerry for complicated reasons of her own. Yet she had to do *something.* So what she did was a displacement, a substitute action. This is the final piece of the puzzle: *Every addictive act is a substitute for a more direct behavior.* This fact leads to one of the important parts of a modern treatment of addiction: If addicts can learn to address their rage at helplessness directly, then it manifests simply as an assertive act. When people act directly, there can be no addiction.

Marion provided a very clear example as she and I worked through her feelings. One day she came in for an appointment and told me that Gerry had done the same thing again—called in the middle of the day to tell her to make dinner for business guests that evening. She said, "I know now what I should have done. I should have told him he could make his own damn dinner. But I just couldn't, so I agreed. The next thing I know, I was going to get my pills." She looked at me and grinned. "But I didn't take any!" It turned out that she found another way: "I knew I had to do something about the damned dinner. Then I thought of it: I called up a Chinese restaurant and ordered take-out." She laughed. "And you know what? As soon as I decided to order the food, my urge to take the pills totally vanished."

Marion's solution wasn't perfect; she knew that the best thing clearly would have been to stand up to her husband. But ordering Chinese food was far more direct than taking Percodan, and the insight that allowed her to understand why she had the urge to take her pills would eventually lead her to defeat her addiction permanently.

As a final side note, this model of addiction also explains why people are able to switch addictions so readily from alcohol to gambling to sex and so on. Although different "addictions" may appear to be wholly separate problems, they are, in fact, just different outward manifestations of the same mechanism. This awareness is often extremely helpful for people as they switch from one addictive focus to the other. Instead of believing they have several diagnoses, they can simply note that the focus of their need to reverse helplessness has changed. (One wonders how this perspective might have helped Bill Wilson, who famously beat drinking, but struggled for the remainder of his life with sexual and smoking compulsions.)

HOW TO TREAT ADDICTION

Understanding the psychological contours of addiction also provides a road map for how to treat it. No longer is it necessary to adopt special spiritual beliefs or join a cohort of people who all suffer with the same problem. Unlocking addiction brings it back down to earth. The problem becomes ordinary, no more or less manageable than any psychological challenge; it needs no special category; it is a psychological problem and can be managed as such.

People who have this symptom can learn how it works within them and develop the agility to solve the issues that lie behind it. For instance, once people view their addiction as a mechanism to solve feelings of overwhelming helplessness, then it becomes critical to identify what is overwhelming for them—what sort of events or feelings carry powerful emotional significance. Being stuck on a call with the bank is frustrating for everybody, but for someone who used to spend hours every week as a child waiting to speak to his estranged father by phone, it carries a particular resonance and power.

Addictive thoughts are never random. To unlock this puzzle, addicts must focus on when the addictive thought first appears. This is the key moment, the pivot point on which everything else turns. By analyzing what happened immediately before this moment—what was just felt or just thought—they can shine a light on the central issue. Yes, each moment is different, and no two people are the same. But we can be certain that they all have something in common: a unifying theme of helplessness about particular issues that are crucial to them. Anyone can learn to recognize these issues for him or herself. Once known, they become far easier to master. People find that they can pause and develop perspective on what is happening. Marion, for instance, knew that her problem was being excessively meek, and this allowed her to pause long enough to understand why she suddenly had the urge to take her pills. Once she realized what was happening, she was able to devise a more direct action to deal with the helplessness. She also gradually found that she could anticipate when the next addictive urge would occur, because she knew what circumstances led to these feelings.

There is always a more direct response to helplessness; this is the lesson to be learned from understanding addictive acts as displacements. It would be beyond the scope of this book to describe all the different ways helplessness can manifest and all the ways people can address these feelings in constructive ways (but many examples can be found in *Breaking Addiction*).[13] For now I will simply say that addiction can be understood, managed, and ended through learning about oneself. People can do a lot on their own, but it is often faster and more helpful to explore these kinds of underlying issues with a professional. For working out these issues permanently, a good psychotherapy is the best approach.

Understanding the nature of addiction helps us clarify why AA, and AA-based rehab programs, have had such limited success. Programs that apply community-based encouragement and little or no individualized care are poorly designed to treat emotional symptoms, including addictive behaviors. It is also easy to see why activities like massage, horses, lectures, and yacht trips don't seem to make much of a dent either. Like the TB sanitaria of the late nineteenth century, 12-step treatments are trying their best to solve a problem whose fundamental essence they do not understand. The fact that a small percentage of people nonetheless become devoted members of 12-step approaches and do well, therefore, raises an interesting question. As we will see in chapter 7, this phenomenon actually makes perfect sense through the prism of a psychological understanding of addiction.

CHAPTER SIX

WHAT THE ADDICTS SAY

THE ACCOUNTS IN THIS CHAPTER tell us a few things about what works and what fails in 12-step treatment, and why. As part of the process of writing this book, I invited (through my blog on *Psychology Today*) firsthand accounts, both positive and negative, of readers' experiences with 12-step programs.[1] This book's writing deadline and space requirements limited the number of interviews I could conduct as well as the total number of accounts that could be included. There was no selection process in choosing the narratives in this chapter; they are simply the reports of the first ten people who responded and gave permission to use their stories in the book. After the deadline I received a number of further accounts; except for a couple of deeply negative reports of people's 12-step experiences, they were remarkable in citing the same combination of positive and negative factors seen in the stories below. These reports tell us much about AA that most people don't hear in popular media.

All of the accounts that follow were either e-mailed or recorded from a telephone interview (each is marked accordingly). The participants gave their permission to use all or any part of their accounts in this book. Their stories have been edited for clarity; some portions were shortened, and material that was deemed repetitive or irrelevant was omitted. Where a person left off a part of his or her views about a topic, then returned to them later, the portions have generally been combined. Except for some minor grammatical fixes, words added for ease of reading have been placed in brackets.

———

ALAN (INTERVIEW)

I grew up in an alcoholic family. My parents were both pretty affluent and successful, but had their own problems. And of course they used alcohol, I think, to suppress themselves. I grew up in a pretty repressed—emotionally repressed—household. . . .

I ended up becoming a single parent by the time I was about twenty-three. By the time my son was about seven, I hadn't been drinking, actually, for a number of years, trying to be a good parent. But I was smoking pot. And, you know, I smoked enough pot, and certainly all my friends were very heavy into drugs, alcohol, hard drugs, soft drugs, everything. So they thought even I was a bit of a lightweight.

But when my son was about seven, I started going to NA, just to try and explore my own drug use, to make sure I wasn't being bad. I certainly wanted to be a good parent to my son, and didn't want to be a bad daddy, doing drugs in front of him. About my first or second NA meeting—which is apparently, I guess, the rule—this guy recruited me to go to rehab—or solicited me. I went to this place in Toronto . . . that wanted to send me to a rehab. . . . They showed me all these lovely pictures of the cottages on the Pacific, so I said, "Sure, I'll sign up for that," because the Ontario health insurance program would pay for it. It was quite expensive, as I recall. Maybe like $30,000 for a twenty-eight-day stay. . . .

I felt entrapped when I got there, because the first thing they do is grab your wallet and say, "You're not getting this back until after twenty-eight days." And they very much threatened me, saying, "If you don't complete the program, you can walk home, because we won't give you a plane ticket back home." I felt kind of coerced, absolutely. . . . But I thought, "It's fine. It's a crash course in psychology, and it'll teach me something, whether it's applicable to me or not" . . . because up to that point, I was four years without a drink.

But when I was there, they constantly hammered me with "You're an alcoholic." And I'm like, "Well, I haven't had a drink in four years. I don't even want a drink. I don't know how you people think I'm an alky." . . . They said it didn't matter. Anybody who has any drug addiction is automatically also an alcoholic. . . . Insofar as I said my parents were alcoholics, they [the counselors] said, "Well, you're automatically alcoholic then, too." That was the extent of their advice. As soon as I said that I didn't agree, they said, "Nope, the argument is this, and until you accept that fact, we have nothing else to talk about." They weren't willing to talk about anything else. . . .

Treatment there was mostly group. I complained long and loud that I wasn't getting any individual therapy and I wanted to talk to someone. So they sent out a psychologist. I spoke to him about three times. He did some sort of a psychological profile on me, and then I had to speak to the psychiatrist who was resident in the facility. She looked at the report, and then—in a rather disgusted way—said to me, "You are anti-authoritarian and antisocial." I thought, wow, that's a hell of a judgment to throw at me. She seemed quite angry about it, and it was very confrontational. I was, like, I don't think this is really helping anything. It may be partially true, but I'm here to work on that stuff, not to get beaten up about it.

Anyway, I did the twenty-eight days . . . and I really enjoyed meeting the people there. Even the nurses' aides were awesome guys to talk to. So that was good. . . . But I could never really hook into the NA and AA philosophy. It seemed forced to me. Oh, and I'll tell you the other thing. I mean, the doctors were always hammering us with a moral side to drug addiction. They seemed really obsessed with religion.

[When] I went back home, I laid off for a while. I didn't smoke for at least thirty days, or sixty days, afterwards. [But] everybody I would meet and befriend in an NA meeting, or even in the odd AA meeting—turned out to be pretty hypocritical. That was kind of hard to take, because they talk a good talk, but they don't walk it. I was grateful for the new friendships, but . . . I haven't been able to retain any friendships in the long term out of any of those experiences, unfortunately. I mean, I wished it was otherwise.

I tried to look at the Twelve Steps and follow what they call a program, but even within the program, people have conflicting opinions. And submitting to a Higher Power seemed kind of illogical to me. It seemed like they were trying to force beliefs on me that I wasn't willing or ready to accept—and kind of contrary to myself. I could see maybe . . . step 4, self-examination, is a good thing, but it seems so religious and dogmatic that it just wasn't effective for me. I couldn't see why they were trying to force beliefs on me that just seemed contrary to common sense, or my experience.

I stopped going to NA [and] AA. I just continued to read on my own about drug addiction and alcoholism, and tried to continue to want to learn from other sources what they were saying, because I really had to dismiss the 12-step dogma. I just couldn't run with it.

I just wanted to be a good father. I wanted to be healthy. I thought, maybe I have to quit smoking in order to be a better person. [But] I was able to accept moderation.

Over the last couple of years I allowed myself to be a moderate drinker, a moderate smoker, without feeling any guilt or compunction about it. I'm a nail-biter. And I realized, every time I'm putting my nails in my mouth it's an emotional reaction. It's not a physical thing. I'm, like, "Your nails are in your face because you feel stressed." I thought, "What's bugging you?" And pretty soon I stopped chewing my nails, and then I stopped wanting to drink, and then the last thing—I guess, in the end—is the marijuana smoking. And I'm, like, "If every time you're putting a drug to your face, you have to stuff your emotions, then why don't you just deal with your emotions and not have to keep stuffing pot in your face?"

I'll have to learn to deal with myself without anything to support me emotionally. . . . I've heard casually from a few psychologists, I guess, but as soon as I hear them espousing 12-step philosophy to me, I'm like, "That's not going to work for me." So I don't even bother.

DIANE (WRITTEN ACCOUNT)

In my personal experience, I was put off immediately by self-demeaning statements that people in AA almost worshipped, statements such as "keep it simple, stupid." Also the vague conflicted religious insinuations.

I was coming out of a difficult relationship, and because he joined AA, I did too. I just wanted to still fit into his life.

My first experience with AA was about ten years ago. A close friend of mine at the time asked me to go to a meeting with her shortly after her mother's death. I went with her. The group consisted mostly of men in their sixties, I think, all of them very disheveled and lost. I don't know if she went back to that particular meeting but she continued with her AA "training."

Another woman I met later, when I was attending meetings myself, has been in the program for twenty-eight years now, I gave her her twenty-five-year chip. Toward the end of my presence in AA, she was feeling unworthy because she could not get out of bed for three weeks and did not attend meetings. The answer that everyone gave her at the meeting, including her sponsor, was that she did not do enough commitments. Commitments in AA mean showing up early and making a pot of coffee or something similar to that. I told her that she [needed] to see a psychiatrist, and she did.

I visited her about two months ago, and she was very different from the severely clinically depressed woman I knew before. She had clinical depression and was guilt-tripped by AA that she was not participating enough. For twenty-five years.

JAMES (WRITTEN ACCOUNT)

I was a homeless addict and drunk for many years, and I got off the streets to go to a community college. I tried AA for five years, and I feel it did more harm than good. AA convinced me that I couldn't drink one drink, and that if I did, that my alcoholic disease would take control of me so that I couldn't stop drinking and that I would die that way. I was scared into staying with AA for a long time. I eventually sought my own answers by majoring in psychology as an undergrad. I came to the conclusion that AA was doing more harm to me, so I left AA and I became ten times more fulfilled than I ever felt in AA. I gained longer sober time, and I eventually came to oppose the disease theory and AA in my life. I am now a very satisfied participant in moderate drinking.

I knew next to nothing when I began attending AA. After attending AA for over a year, I began to believe many of the things that were stated repeatedly at meetings. I came to believe that I had no willpower over a powerful disease and that the only thing that could save me was lifelong AA attendance along with extreme commitment and service to the AA program. At this point, I felt trapped by a cult that held a mysterious solution to alcohol addiction. I believed what AA told me and that was that I would die from alcoholism without AA or that I would be a bitter miserable dry drunk the rest of my life. I believed the idea, pushed by AA and the powers that be that push AA, that even one drink meant that I was not recovered or in a relapse. In retrospect, I realize that these beliefs pushed by AA were harmful to me because it caused me to seriously believe I had no willpower to stop drinking, which led to numerous drinking binges that lasted up to five days at a time every couple of weeks or so. The fear of harming others during a binge and terrible legal and financial consequences related to drinking were other factors that kept me fearful and dependent on the AA program.

After sixteen months of not being in AA, I now believe I have the internal locus of control to moderate my drinking. Since leaving AA, I have found numerous websites and stories of the things I felt [were] wrong in AA but that I had no words for at the time. . . . I continue to find people sympathetic to alternatives to the traditional 12-step disease model fixated on abstinence.

Going to AA for five years was not all for nothing . . . because those actions (cleaning up before and after meetings, making coffee, etc.) were my personal actions showing my personal commitment, energy, and discipline to living a healthier life. [But] AA socialization also prevented me from growing as much as I should have otherwise. Everything I did revolved around AA principles, so many important issues had been neglected and not discussed in my life during those five years.

While in AA, there was only room for complete bias in favor of AA. In fact, I had hoped that confessing about how great AA was and about how AA saved me would somehow help "the miracle" happen and that I was "faking it till I made it"—which are AA slogans. Well, the miracle never happened in AA, and I no longer depend on whatever mystery people claim exists in AA. I felt AA was veiled by mystery, which also kept me going for five years. The closest person to me, my mother, said that I have improved tremendously since leaving AA. My mother said that while in AA I seemed to be in a severe state of agitation. She says that now I am much more the person she has always known from even before I ever used drugs or alcohol. I even feel that I am more *me* rather than an alcoholic so and so from AA.

I had a negative experience with AA, but professionally I believe I will have to be more objective and balanced in giving the pros and cons of AA with others and how it might work for them. I believe I lay out so many cons to AA because the treatment industry seems to blindly promote all the pros of AA.

SHARON (WRITTEN ACCOUNT)

Twenty-two years ago, my high school sweetheart died. He struggled with addiction but he had more than ninety days clean when he died. He had a good job and his life was finally on track for a bright future. He went to meetings. We talked of marriage and children. He was working "the steps" and had recently found a "sponsor." Everything was going well.

He started to pay people back money he had borrowed under false pretenses, which he had used to buy drugs. He bought his sister tickets to a concert because at some point in the past she had missed one and he felt it had been his fault. He donated time and money to charities. His family was thrilled to see this.

I worried. I couldn't exactly say why. Something just seemed off. When I brought up how changed he seemed, how he seemed almost frantic about doing these things, I was told not to worry. He seemed really down, I was told that was related to his recovery, that it was a good thing. He was making "amends." He was "working the steps." His family and a few of his new friends from AA all suggested that I look into Al-Anon.

It was a Friday. We were having dinner with his mom and sister. I thought he was picking me up after he got off work. When he didn't call and didn't show up, I just thought I misunderstood the plan so I went over to his Mom's. He never showed up. They figured he had relapsed. The next morning I called a few of his friends. No one had heard from him.

My heart stopped when I heard the knock on my door. Something about the quick loud rap alarmed me. Two uniformed officers were at my door. I don't remember what they asked me or anything they said. Except that my sweetheart was dead. He was clean when he died. He hung himself.

How has AA impacted my life? AA prevented my sweetheart's family from recognizing the warning signs for suicide for what they were. When I expressed concern about what he was doing, it was dismissed. [I was told] my problem was I didn't know enough about how AA works—I didn't go to Al-Anon meetings or read the literature.

It is true. I didn't understand how AA worked, I had not read the literature. When I did, I found it very troubling. It is easy to see how the warning signs for suicide were missed or dismissed. Admit you are powerless, take a moral inventory, make amends. Steps. A sense of powerlessness, attempts to settle debts . . . isolating from family and friends. Suicide warning signs.

JEN (WRITTEN ACCOUNT)

I asked to go to rehab after a stint in the hospital. One night I had gotten pulled over for driving on the wrong side of the highway. . . . They sent me to the hospital instead of taking me to jail. I don't know how that happened, but I got really lucky and, you know, my luck was running out. So my dad came and picked me up from the hospital the next morning. I hadn't known what happened and I asked to go to rehab. So I went to rehab for about five weeks. I learned a lot there, it was great. Then they recommended that I go to a step-down care house, kind of like a halfway house. So I did that.

I stuck with the 12-step meetings, and whatnot, for about my first year of sobriety. I became really close with the woman that wound up becoming my sponsor. But she started treating me like her daughter, because I reminded her of her daughter. And after about a year, every time I went to a meeting, it didn't work for me. I mean, I'm still sober. I don't even like saying that I'm sober. It's just, it's my life; I just made a decision to not drink. And I think it's kind of a cult and they kind of set you up to relapse. It's not fair that they put all these thoughts into your head where if you leave the community they make you believe that that sets you up for a relapse, because you no longer have that community and that support network available to you. They say, we'll always welcome you back. Then when people come back they say they relapsed because they stopped going to meetings. It's not that they stopped going to meetings. They started isolating themselves and they let problems get to their head.

You'll ask kids that go in and out of the rooms why they went out and relapsed and they just say, "I stopped going to meetings." I don't think that that's the case whatsoever. I actually feel a lot better now that I stopped going, because I feel like I'm putting my ego down, saying I'm an alcoholic or an addict. I've chosen not to drink, I saw where it took me in life, and I've been, quote-unquote, "sober" for about two and a half years now, and I'm only twenty-four. So the way I see it, all you really need is a support network and a drive to want to continue making yourself a better person.

They say, "One day at a time," and when you start feeling really crummy come to a meeting and complain about it and you'll get support from other people. And I just think it's silly. . . . I mean, I can't even really remember a lot of the things that they say in the 12-step meetings, because I just don't apply those to my life anymore, because I've kind of learned things on my own. I mean the only step I really, really did was, I made a fearless moral inventory of myself. That's really the only one I got anything out of, to be honest. Because I sat down, I talked to the woman that had gotten really close with me, my sponsor. But anytime they brought up the word God, I just got up and walked away. Because religion is like politics to me, I just don't believe in it. AA is more kind of old-school in the sense where they talk about God a lot more. And you have to say the Lord's Prayer, and whatnot. At the rehab, they didn't talk to you about AA so much, they just talked to you about what you said, about meditating and getting to be at one with yourself.

I understood what they said about the spiritual stuff. But it's just like there's only certain beliefs you can stick to when you're in that program. Like the fact that you have to still admit you're an alcoholic or a drug addict. You have to have a Higher Power. I'm kind of looking at the steps right now to kind of remember. This stuff was literally like my form of religion when I used to go to it. But it frustrates me now. I just find it annoying. But I still, you know, if I talk to people that are still in recovery or "newcomers," quote-unquote, I say, "Stick with it, it does a lot for you at first, because you have that network and you see that you're not alone." But you get to a certain point where you don't want to be around those people anymore. I mean, if you stick in the rooms long enough, you see people go in and out of there at least once a week.

PAUL (INTERVIEW)

In my mind, I didn't really get sober in AA. I think to get sober in AA would be really difficult because often, but not always, I've seen newcomers just be completely ignored at the end of meetings. So, I always try to make it a point to go up and give my phone number. But most of them will rarely call me, because there's no structure around working with newcomers; it's very easy to fall through the cracks, and I think that's what happens with the majority of people that come into AA.

Obviously, AA has its benefits. It gives you a place to go. I met a lot of close friends. I went to meetings every day for years, and I liked it. At first, I felt like it was a cult, but then I decided it was my cult, you know, and I could kind of do what I'd want, and sort of ran a meeting. I liked doing that. I was pretty happy with AA until the bottom dropped out, emotionally, and I fell into a very severe depression, and then nobody wanted to hear my story, because the narrative is: you drink, your life falls apart, you go to AA, you stop drinking, your life gets better. And that wasn't my narrative.

I received a lot of negativity, a lot of criticism from people, even from people with much less sober time than me. They told me that I wasn't doing the steps correctly because I was discussing how I felt. People would actually get up and walk out when I started talking, since I was saying things about how I felt. It makes some intellectual sense to me that they try to keep conversation on the solution, rather than the problem, but . . . my problem was the dark mood that I was experiencing.

I've been sober over twenty years. I've tried various times to go back to AA, just to have some friends, but I just found it difficult. I lived in southern California, then after maybe six, seven years of sobriety, I lived in New York City, and I found the AA meetings there to be especially militant. People would immediately ask you who your sponsor was, and what's your home group, and they wanted to run your program. You've probably heard the phrase, "taking somebody's inventory." That's done as a matter of course, and I found it to be offensive. So I didn't really like meetings there very much. I would go, and I would feel worse. Eventually, I realized that going to AA was, like, the worst: the meetings made me feel bad, and

I felt that the conversation was a little superficial. People were expected to solve their [problems], make their life better, and it didn't fit reality.

My other pet peeve with AA is the whole sponsorship thing. . . . I sensed a dynamic very often where you get into a hierarchical relationship, because they kind of see themselves as guiding you. It's not a peer relationship. And many of these people, while they mean well, they're just not qualified to be giving advice to the degree that they are. And I've heard a lot of sponsors try to hide the truth of their life from their sponsees, because they don't want to be seen as flawed and human. The whole thing is kind of silly to me, and I know that there are ways to work with people without getting into that relationship. But I should say, the first sponsor relationship I had was very helpful to me; I had somebody who I could call, and he would understand me. But I found a therapist that said, "You need to be on Prozac" . . . [and] that ended my relationship with my sponsor, and his lineage: his sponsor, [who was] like a grand sponsor . . . and some old guy, who had thirty years sobriety or something. They all decided that I was basically taking drugs.

After I came out of treatment . . . AA helped me not drink because I really had, at that point, very little social structure in place, and it . . . gave me a support network. I can only remember one or two times where I really, really wanted to drink . . . and, you know, it's hard to say what I would've done had I not had that support network, but I certainly think it made things easier emotionally to have that, especially in early sobriety. The thing about AA that's good is people are very honest about their experience, and that's an honesty that is not common in our society. So, that sharing I think can really strengthen your own sort of emotional self.

[As for] the steps, I got something out of doing the confessional step. That felt very cathartic to me, and I know that a lot of spiritual traditions [have] a similar mechanism in place. So I definitely got something out of that, and the meditative practice step [step 11] is good. [But] the God part was a big turnoff. In fact, I had been on hard drugs previously, and . . . I went to an NA meeting, and . . . I might have gotten sober or clean at that point, except at the end of the meeting, they all stood around and said the Lord's Prayer, and it's Catholic, and I'm not interested in that charade. So I didn't go back. In fact, I've traveled across the country and been to meetings where everyone in the meeting was a born-again Christian and felt like you needed to get Jesus before you get sober. So I certainly wouldn't have been able to hang in meetings in those localities.

CHERYL (INTERVIEW)

For many reasons I drank quite heavily for about seventeen years. Circumstances in my life brought me to a point where I went into therapy, a psychoanalytical therapy. I'd been in therapy for about two and a half years, and my therapist was telling me that my therapy wasn't progressing very well because whenever I had an insight I'd drink it away. [Then] I had kind of a psychological breakthrough—I had a memory that surfaced, that I couldn't drink away. I realized that I needed to stop drinking.

I went to my first AA meeting. I really didn't like the religious aspect of it at all, because I'd come from an evangelical background, and the whole God thing made me really angry. . . . [But] everybody was very supportive instead of being condemning. And my friends told me that it was a program of honesty. I couldn't tolerate the meetings much more than one a week for the first year, which is really tough for somebody who's recovering from alcoholism. But I went to therapy every week . . . [and] I stayed at the meetings because it was the only place where I felt like I could, with other people, be honest. And that's pretty much why I stayed with Alcoholics Anonymous.

I've been continuously sober for nineteen years, but there've been some years when I haven't gone. I chose to end my relationship with my parents, and because of the spiritual focus of the program, I knew there were some people who would tell me that I should just let God heal the relationship. And I couldn't tolerate that. And honestly . . . the one great thing about AA is every time I go and somebody only has a day or two or a week or two or a month or two, it does reinforce my desire not to drink and go back there. Really. It reinforces that. But there are other aspects of AA—they tell you, as you all know, when you first came in that you can't say no to a request. And then it took me several years to learn that yes, I can say no . . . to, like, a request to speak or do service work. And I think that's particularly true with women in AA. They come in very codependent, and it takes a while to learn how to set boundaries and say no. And some AA meetings are

supportive of that and some are not. Like most people in AA, I came in . . .
I didn't know how to relate to other people. And I tended to pick the most
dysfunctional people in the room. A lot of newcomers pick people who are
kind of where they are. And it's a painful thing to learn that not everybody
in the room is safe, not everybody in the room is healthy, and not everybody in the room has your best interests at heart. They can be 13th-stepping
[taking advantage of another member sexually or financially]. Some people
are sicker than others. And I think AA works best if someone's in therapy.
But that's not a traditional AA approach.

I think for the first six months to a year, everything is so raw and so,
depending on how much alcohol you consumed and for how long, most
people's nerves are shot and their relationships are shot and usually their
finances are shot. It's really nice to be in a room full of people who understand what a big mess you have. The only problem is that after six months
or a year of drying out and making a few better choices, what I've found is
a lot of my family of origin patterns and a lot of bad habits of interrelating
with people surfaced, and I can take the same language of AA and justify
those same old patterns of behavior. A lot of what I thought of as being a
good AA person was really me acting out a whole lot of my people-pleasing
nature. I wanted everybody in the room to like me, so I didn't question
what they said. That can get you in some odd situations and weird relationships, depending on who's in the room with you.

So much of AA depends on who your sponsor is. Those relationships,
when people are coming out of alcohol addiction, become just incredibly
important. You can choose the wrong people, and it can be a car wreck. It's
potluck who you get; it's potluck who comes to a meeting.

I don't think alcohol is the problem. I think alcohol is the symptom.
What I've seen in my own life, and also in AA, is you stop drinking but you
tend to act out compulsively other places. The smoking, the caffeine, eating, sex, gambling. The addiction switches.

One of the things I've never seen any studies on is, I think I've probably known five to ten people who've killed themselves in AA . . . just in the
years I've gone. My sponsor killed himself . . . and four or five people who
go to this same meeting have died by killing themselves. This is why a lot
of people I know, in their third or fourth year, go into therapy, some kind

of therapy. Because they understand that being sober is not solving every-thing. If they're lucky, they go into some kind of therapy.

[In] AA, people don't care if you're in therapy, [but] some people do care if you take prescription drugs around mental problems. The weird thing about AA is there is no organization. Every group is autonomous. Every group sets their own standards. The reason I stay with the group that I go to is we have a lot of therapists, we have a lot of priests, we have a lot of social workers in it. So they have a different perspective than if it was a group of people who . . . only have the AA orthodoxy to fall back on. I came from an evangelical Christian point of view, so I'm always very hesitant when people start quoting the Big Book at me. It's like, you know, don't tell me chapter and verse about this. Because I don't believe it's an orthodoxy. AA is definitely a spiritual path. People say you can take God out of it, and a lot of people do. But at that point, you pretty much go to it for a social and a group support network.

I have seen AA not work for everyone for a lot of different reasons. And when you talk about AA, it's one of those nebulous things like saying "the Catholic Church." Some parishes may be really, really great and strong and wonderful with a great priest. And others can be really, really corrupt, with a pedophile. Who knows what you're going to get? That's the bad thing about therapists just telling people to go to AA. They have no idea what they're going to get.

MARTINA (INTERVIEW)

AA is just not for everybody. And when you do come across something in your life that's maybe causing you to have a craving or something like that . . . you're just met with a lot of slogans and things. You know, "One day at a time," or "Work the Twelve Steps harder," "Pray harder." It's never really addressed why you might have these cravings in the first place. So it's really hard to get the help that you need, and it is very rigid. People would share their experiences, but always with the afterthought, "AA saved my life." And then the AA slogans would come in, and everything was credited to AA. They are very rigid and no other options are really offered to you, as to any kind of help you may need.

Young people would come in—very desperate, just clinging to anything that would help them. AA [was] offered as a solution without any other choices or options . . . and they needed other help. It would seem obvious to me, as I got to know them, that there were other things they needed in their life to help them get over whatever reason they were drinking in the first place. And they were struggling. They were distressed. They needed someone to talk to, even if it was just going to their general practitioner or someone who they could talk to and maybe recommend a therapist or a psychiatrist, or whatever they may need at that point. They really needed something like that and they would struggle. Some of them would commit suicide because it became just too much for them. [Then, in the meetings] the impression you would get was that they were pretty much at fault for this, because either they didn't work the program hard enough or go to enough meetings, or they had some kind of character defect that prevented them from working the program right. So, it always basically came down to—these people died because they had this disease of alcoholism or addiction, and they were flawed, and that was just the outcome. I'm sure I wasn't the only one that could see beyond that—that maybe this person could have been saved if they were offered some other kind of treatment. But [some of those who had done well] saw that as the only way. It worked for them for so many years, that that was the answer to everything. It's just the get-tough kind of mentality: "If it isn't working for you, just suck it up. Get tough and work the program, and you'll be fine."

And, talking to a lot of these old-timers, they all had the same drinking patterns through their life. They had been alcoholics for many, many years, and it was a lifestyle. My second sponsor, actually, was one of those old-timers. She had been sober for twenty-five years. She was a good person and she was doing well. I felt bad that she felt the need, after twenty-five years, to still label herself as an alcoholic—that that was what she was, and that she still needed AA. I remember mentioning to her at one time that maybe after twenty-five years, maybe she should take a little credit—you know, "You did a good job. That's great." But she couldn't do that, you know? The only reasons she was sober twenty-five years, in her opinion, was because of AA, and because of God. And without this, she would surely drink again. She really felt that way. And it was, actually, kind of sad.

It seemed like we had a lot of people that were mandated into AA through the court system. But that could be dangerous, I think. I think if someone's in the court system because, maybe, multiple DUIs, I can see where a judge, maybe in frustration, or to try to help the person, would send them to AA. But there were people who, when they got drunk, beat their wives, or molested their kids or something, but they wouldn't do that when they were sober. The judge might mandate them to AA, thinking, well, alcohol is the problem. And that's fine, as long as that person stays sober. But you're in a group of people who know nothing about this person. What if this person shows up drunk or something, or, you know, slips? Then it's kind of dangerous, I think. Something else needs to be done for that person other than sending them to AA.

I was able to work through my own issues. I was able to learn about myself. Not just in therapy, outside of therapy, I could reflect back on my life, and just get to know myself more, and why I did the things I did. I realized that it had nothing to do with character defects or that I had to be humble and be kept down all the time. I could recognize my strengths, too, and where I could grow. And, it was just beneficial all around for me. I do have an occasional drink once in a while. But I came to that conclusion after some therapy, and realizing that, although abstinence certainly is something that some people really should do, for me, it wasn't. I could have a couple of drinks now and again, and I don't have to worry about it continuing, and turning into, maybe, becoming physically dependent on the alcohol again. That never happened to me again, except that one time when I was originally hospitalized.

Inpatient is when they first expose you to an AA meeting. It was a hospital that used the 12-step principles in their therapy, or whatever. And the initial meeting, inpatient, was more an informative kind of meeting—just learning about what AA was, and what it was about kind of thing. But then, in the outpatient rehab that I was doing, we were required to go to three meetings a week, whether it be NA or AA or whatever was appropriate for a person. We were required to get a sponsor, and to at least work through our first step while we were in the program. And that's all that was offered. There was nothing—no other options were ever talked about or offered to anybody.

They will be very adamant about saying this is not a religious program—that it's spiritual in nature, but it is not a religion. But as you read the Twelve Steps, it's very obvious it is a religion. And it tends to be more Christian in nature, I think. And like I said, for me, it wasn't so much of a problem, because I was raised a Christian. I do believe in God. I feel spiritual, and I felt strong enough in my religious beliefs that I didn't have to follow theirs. But it's very strange, you know? It's like you're told, if you don't believe in God, you have to believe in something—some Higher Power. And it could be anything, you know? It could be the group. It could be another person. It could be a doorknob or a rock. I mean, it just seems so ridiculous, and just crazy, you know? I just didn't get that. But it's just the way they took the religion, like they were some separate group. That God saw them differently, somehow, and favored them, and looked upon them favorably, as long as they stayed sober. You know, it was just very strange. I'm just really glad I didn't really fall into that or buy into that. I think, in some cases, that some people had the attitude that as long as they toed the line, followed the rules, that they were in God's favor. You know, God would treat them better.

Honestly, I think [the faith part of AA] could be done without. I don't think it belongs there. It should be a support, and the support-group setting where anyone who has an addiction problem should feel free to come without feeling harassed about their religion. You know, I don't think it's very important. . . . I mean, I would have prayed regardless if I was in AA or not. And people who have that inclination are going to practice their religion or spirituality, anyway. People who don't buy into that, or don't believe in God, or are atheists, or whatever, I don't think should be subjected to this as part of their treatment. They [atheists] do have a separate meeting, and I'm sure it works well for a lot of them. But God is in the Twelve Steps, or at least a Higher Power, so I don't think you'll ever really get away from that.

TOM (WRITTEN ACCOUNT)

After twenty-five years of abstinence from alcohol, I returned drinking five years ago when I retired. The reasons are many and varied. I have never bought into the "disease model." To me, the disease model is a lot of smoke and mirrors. I was abused by my mother and sexually molested by a high school "guidance" counselor. Did these incidents cause me to develop a disease?

I got drunk the first time I ever had my first drink when I was eighteen. This continued for twelve years. I finally quit in 1979 and did not touch liquor or drugs for twenty-five years. People who work in the field of addictions maintain that my addiction was caused by some malfunctioning gene or some other idiotic conundrum, or that I was predisposed to the disease of addiction. Really? How was it that I was able to quit for twenty-five years? Can a cancer patient quit having cancer? Can a diabetic suddenly decide not to be a diabetic any longer? My addiction was a direct result of severe emotional trauma, and my substance abuse was a reaction to blot out my serious mental torment.

During my drinking and drugging days, I had many experiences in "treatment" centers, private counselors and a host of other charlatans all claiming that I had a disease. Treatment centers are, by their very nature, heavily disposed to this convoluted thinking . . . [that] to maintain any type of stability I must get involved in a 12-step program, and it begins even while one is in the hospital.

To further elaborate on my hospital experiences, one instance stands out in particular. In this group, each person is given a large sheet of poster board and then is asked to cut out things from a stack of magazines and paste them on the board while soft relaxing music is playing in the background. At this point, I expected to find myself embroiled in Tinkertoy or Lincoln Log therapy. Then there were the usual group sessions. Each person had a sheet which was to be filled out and shared with the group. As a bit of an aside, the pencils were made of pliable plastic just in case someone in the group went berserk. The counselor would then ask: "How are we feeling today?" "Angry?" "Depressed?" "Happy?" "Sad?" etc. This would be followed by the usual rant session.

Hospitalizations are a total waste of time, and most of the people I spoke with in treatment held the same views. Most people went there to get "dried out" as I did, play the game, get out, and go back to doing what one was doing previously, i.e., drinking or drugging. I cannot imagine the therapists were so oblivious to all this that they really believed that all this nonsense was useful as a part of one's "recovery."

Speaking of recovery, the 12-steppers are always "in recovery"; even if the person has been off the stuff for years, they are still considered to be in recovery. No one ever recovers. Ultimately this leads to dependency on the group rather than on a healthy self-reliance. If I were to state that I used to have an addiction to alcohol, I would be met with hoots of derision from 12-steppers, since total recovery is impossible. Is it any wonder why there is such a lack of success in the treatment industry? One is essentially set up to fail. If one is never to recover, why bother? I believe that there is a method to this madness. It keeps the revolving door constantly revolving and the money keeps rolling in.

Most of the meetings I attended ranged from the mundane to the laughable, since I would often see several of these people walk into a bar immediately after attending a meeting. Some members who usually attended meetings and were suddenly absent were described as being "out there"—meaning, of course, that they went back to drinking or drugging. The comment was often made that his or her disease "got 'em." The "oldtimers"—those with the most abstinence, or who claimed to have the most— were treated with subservience boarding on awe. These people generally ran the meetings. They would often give shopworn speeches about the old days and how they beat demon rum with the help of their "Higher Power." As I was to learn, a higher power could be anything. People said, "Well, it can be anything; you can make a doorknob your Higher Power if you wish as long as you stay clean and sober." A doorknob? This is utter insanity.

After a few years of this nonsense I finally quit drinking because I came to understand the damage I was doing not only to myself but the emotional trauma to my wife, who never knew what she would find when she came home. She knew that I drove drunk and feared that I would either kill myself or some other poor unfortunate who happened to be in the wrong place at the wrong time.

The really sad part of all the "treatment" business is that it is costing taxpayers billions of dollars. Treatment centers are a scam. Individual treatment centers take in hundreds of thousands of dollars annually with little to show for their effort, since many who leave the centers often return to their addictions. But, they are always welcomed back no matter how often.

There is one stipulation: one must have insurance or the available resources to pay out of pocket.

LINDA (WRITTEN ACCOUNT)

To detail my 12-step experience in proper context it is necessary for me to go back to before I ever began drinking alcohol. I am forty-eight years old and grew up in [a small town]. I remember suffering from anxiety problems at a very young age. My mother had me on some kind of tranquilizer the pediatrician prescribed when I was eleven because I would have emotional meltdowns. I recall my first very bad depression, which coincided with the onset of . . . OCD at age twelve (though it would be decades before I would have a name for these intrusive, horrific thoughts). I tried to just make it through these episodes throughout my adolescence. The severity of the obsessional thoughts and accompanying depression would ebb and flow. When the thinking would start, I would lose interest in everything I enjoyed and would reach a point of feeling nothing at all save misery. I made it through these periods and kept good grades and was a well-behaved girl to all who knew me.

My breaking point came at eighteen, when I had an episode so bad that I literally couldn't get out of bed and couldn't stand the sunlight and had to force myself to eat. I asked my parents for psychiatric help and tried to describe my problems. They were ashamed and upset but got me an appointment with a psychiatrist. The psychiatrist I saw didn't seem to understand all my symptoms and gave me a tricyclic antidepressant and told me I shouldn't feel this way, since I had a college scholarship waiting on me. The medication did very little to help me and I got no insight as to what the obsessional thoughts were and how to stop them. I found a way to make the thoughts stop for a short period of time on my own later that summer when I drank most of a fifth of vodka my Dad had bought months ago to mix some drinks for some occasion. Alcohol seemed like my answer. I proceeded to drink the bottle and take every pill I could find in the house, I just wanted as much relief from thinking as I could get. I was sent to the hospital with an overdose. I was sent on to college that fall.

My relationship with my parents became very bad because of my drinking. By the end of my senior year in college, I sought out a psychiatrist again after a breakup with a boyfriend. I entered graduate school in order to prolong my schooling, now I [realize] because I knew in my heart once I entered my chosen profession of teaching, my anxiety levels would skyrocket out of control.

My teaching career was a very short plummet into hell. My anxiety levels were insane, my depression was taking me down, and I was without contact with my previous doctor. I drank heavily to try to manage my out-of-control emotions, and it only took about a year and a half until I was out of a job and drinking hopelessly. I went in and out of psychiatric units for a year and was put on progressively more intense medications . . . though the doctors I saw knew I was drinking. It was a godsend when I finally fell into the hands of two social workers who sent me to detox and then got me an indigent bed in a twenty-one-day treatment center. My parents were through with me; I had nothing and no one.

I experienced AA for the first time in that treatment center. They would take us to meetings. I had never smoked but I wanted to fit into this group of people so badly I began buying cigarettes. My counselor at the treatment center was a very kind man who was a recovering alcoholic also. It was recommended that I go on to [a rehab] for long-term treatment of about a year. I was happy to do this, since I had nothing and people in the treatment and AA world were treating me humanely.

[At the rehab] there seemed to me to be a very hard push to get people to see sexual abuse in their backgrounds. At the time it seemed that the assumption was that a woman had to have been sexually abused to be an alcoholic. I always felt like they thought I was lying when I told them I was not.

When I left [there] after a year I was going to very many meetings per week. I had a job by then at a factory and all I did was work and go to AA meetings. In fact, I basically did that for years. I didn't know what to do with myself for a very long time if I had spare time and wasn't at a meeting; I felt very guilty because people said if you slacked off meetings you would get drunk.

It was about this time that I heard old-timers talk about people not really being sober if they were on psychiatric medications. I had been on Tegretol and Elavil at the [rehab], but had asked the psychiatrist . . . there if I could stop taking these. I didn't want to feel like my sobriety could be called into question by anyone, and I also mistrusted psychiatric medication at this point and believed my only problem ever was that I had been an alcoholic (pre-alcoholic before I drank). The psychiatrist said that was fine. I only ever saw this lady [the psychiatrist] once when I entered the [rehab] and again just before I left. No one seemed to consider ongoing problems like depression, anxiety, or anything else unless these crept up in some way that disturbed the calm of the [rehab], then that person would go to a psych hospital for a week and get meds, or a change in meds.

I really worried quite a bit about someone questioning my [sober] "time." I used to worry that a particular local AA matriarch would want me to say I had a year less "time" if she knew I had been on medication when I was in long-term treatment. I obsessed on this. She used to refer to women who were on antidepressants as "Prozac babies" and said that they couldn't feel enough pain to work the steps properly on medication. I also was terribly afraid of being yelled at in a meeting. I didn't like to share in meetings because I had seen old-timers yell at people and I had seen people use non-AA phrasing and be shot down and humiliated. One time, when I was a couple of years sober, I was at a meeting and a group of people from a local treatment center were brought to the meeting. One woman introduced herself as an "addict," and all kinds of rage broke loose from the old-timers at the meeting. The person who brought the group left the meeting and the rest of the meeting was spent with people talking about how that was the only way to handle it. Those incidents were frightening. I lived in fear of being humiliated and getting drunk over it.

Looking back, I was rather lucky in one way when I got sober. I was overweight from the mix of meds I had been given over time and I was working a minimum-wage job. This did not make me attractive to men in the AA meetings I was attending. There were some women I lived with at the [rehab] who were very attractive though, and they were basically harassed by men as if they were merchandise to be obtained. They would get so many phone calls that they would stop coming to the phone. It was disgusting. [The rehab] did not like for any of us to date during our first year, but these ladies were chased by men. I had never seen grown men behave the way they did in AA.

There is such reverence given to "time" in AA—especially to those who have time and have a huge following of sponsees or started a meeting or some such—that it skews the actual aims of "recovery" in my opinion. Certain people can't be questioned, even when they do questionable things, and humiliating people in meetings becomes "telling them like it is." There is a certain AA arrogance that exists, one that assumes we "drunks" can only understand each other, the doctors and psychiatrists can never help us. I bought into some of this, but not the cult of personality. I avoided meetings that were run by particular old-timers or those that were very fundamentalist in the way they approached the Twelve Steps.

I saw a fundamentalist strain coming into being when I was about two to three years sober, and these people frightened me worse than the old-timers. In their philosophy, you must do the steps perfectly or you will get drunk. These people always look back on everything that they ever had happen, even as a child, and say it was their "selfishness and self-centered fear" and it showed that they were just an alcoholic. They have a very smooth way of speaking. . . . I have steered clear of groups like this.

I made sure to pick a very benign sponsor. I knew I would not be accepted fully in the AA community without one, and I had to have one when I lived at the [rehab]. I had a great fear of sponsorship; my relationship with my mother has never been good and I did not want some other woman controlling my life. Unfortunately this is what sponsorship is in many cases. Women especially are conditioned in AA to be very hard on themselves. I felt pressure from the first time I spoke about my past at a meeting at the [rehab] to make sure to not "blame" anyone else for anything that happened to me, to focus on it being because of my alcoholism. A person learns to tell their story in the way that others will find acceptable. I feel, and I have heard it in other women's "stories" an unspoken pressure to . . . shame myself to a certain extent. There was a point where I wondered if I was really telling the truth anymore after years of this.

There is an ideal that [if] you have any negative emotion about anything, then you are the person at fault. If you are harmed by someone else then you are at fault for being around them, if something bad happens to you then WHY NOT YOU, you are an alcoholic. I once heard a woman discuss . . . how she read an amends letter at the grave of a man who had sexually abused her as a child. I was very upset by hearing that a sponsor told her to do such a thing. Sponsors often act like some combination of therapist and parent and are not qualified to be a therapist and should not parent an adult!

I had a woman ask me to sponsor her a few years ago after her previous sponsor, upon being told she had drunk again, went into a screaming rage on the woman. She was so verbally beaten down by that sponsor that after a few months in AA she told me that she just didn't feel safe in AA and did not return. I don't blame her. This was a fear I had in the beginning, that I would be on the receiving end of someone's screaming, raging, insults, and humiliation. AA has to be the only place where completely uncivilized behavior is not only accepted but often applauded. The victim will nearly always be asked what their part was, in effect putting all blame squarely on their shoulders.

Along the way I met a man in AA and we got married. We are still married. There are strong opinions in AA on whether or not someone should or should not marry a fellow member. I know that for me, making a life with someone I feel like I really can trust has been the right decision. I've seen others hurt greatly in relationships with fellow AA members.

Throughout eighteen years of my sobriety, I worked hard to try to at least hide my roller-coaster emotions, anxiety, OCD, and off-and-on depression. When my father passed away, I made a decision to seek medical treatment for my depression and anxiety. It was like a veil of misery lifted. My mental health is not perfect but I am so much better that I began to wonder if the exalted Twelve Steps ever did anything for me besides grant me membership into a group of people who at least didn't see me as worthless. I had run across criticism of AA online here and there and had paused to read it, agreeing with many of the complaints others had. Now I read all I could get, I went all through the Orange Papers [an online site critical of

AA] in an afternoon, feeling relief in so much of it. I really think that the moralistic tone of the Twelve Steps is at best outdated, and at worst next to useless.

I do give old-timers, now gone, credit for one thing: they did not push a Christian God at newcomers. The ones I knew took the idea of "a power greater than yourself" seriously and did not rush anyone to decide how they approached it. Now I hear more religiosity in the tone. . . . A problem with AA's idea of a "God as you understand him" is that the program goes on to tell you exactly how to pray, and many people in AA will insist you get on your knees to humble yourself before God. This is hardly in keeping with the idea of "how you understand." This has to be quite off-putting to believers and non-believers alike in many cases, and should be. The way the Big Book describes agnostics is very belittling.

I can read the Big Book now and see many parts that are not myself. Bill Wilson made assumptions about the "alcoholic personality" that members of AA are demanded to identify themselves with that I do not believe are true in all, or even most, cases. This is grossly unfair and unhelpful. So much homage is paid to the "Big Book," and I no longer believe much of it stands up to actual research or even observable reality. Look at some poor person who suffers from an undiagnosed mental illness drinking to self-medicate, [do you] tell them they have an "ego problem" and can't recover until their ego is smashed?

I still attend one meeting a week . . . [and] I love the people at the AA meeting I attend, but when I am in a meeting I hear many things and think, "That's not really true; we just have to say that in AA." I think AA would be a much better organization without its literature. There has to be a better way to help alcoholics. I needed medication for so long but was led to believe my alcoholic status negated that need. Once declared an alcoholic, that became the only problem professionals made any real attempts at helping me with. People need to be willing to actually look at what works and doesn't work in treating drug and alcohol problems. I think a lot of people are suffering needlessly because they can't learn to speak AA and live in the AA culture overnight; I think not "getting" this contrived culture is called denial and people are abandoned by AA and by treatment professionals because of it.

COMMENTARY

The above accounts indicate that AA's strength lies in providing a social network where newly abstinent people can get together comfortably in mutual support. But their stories also reflect some of AA's serious problems. AA is ungoverned by design, which means it can also be unpredictable and unreliable: there is no consistent quality control. Some meetings are run by mature and thoughtful people, others by unsophisticated fundamentalists. You might get warm and avuncular advice, or you might find yourself on the receiving end of a personally driven, hurtful rant.

These stories also underscore another problem of 12-step programs: misdiagnosis. It is a common belief in AA that if you have alcoholism, all your troubles in life and any psychological issues with which you suffer are also "alcoholism." Emboldened by an outsized confidence that they know what's right for people with addictions, many in AA believe they are competent to make such assessments. It is startling that professionals who would never prescribe a drug whose contents were unreliable or send people with emotional symptoms to untrained laymen nonetheless regularly send people to 12-step meetings.

These case studies also highlight one place where AA could do a better job. We have already seen the statistical research indicating that many people dislike the religious nature of AA; these stories underscore just how personal that disillusionment can be. Someone who wanted to design a peer support network for addicts today would be wise to eliminate all vestiges of AA's fundamentalist roots. This would mean discarding nearly all of the Twelve Steps except for step 4: self-examination. As these accounts show, many addicts note the value of this concept, which makes sense, since self-understanding is the key to treating all psychological symptoms. Unfortunately, AA's version of this—the "fearless moral inventory"—is sullied by its moralistic character. Since the goal of therapy is to help people recognize feelings and thoughts that lie beyond their awareness, every good psychotherapist must avoid the mistake of imposing a moral agenda.

CHAPTER SEVEN

WHY DOES AA WORK WHEN IT DOES?

AS WE HAVE SEEN, the overall success rate of AA lies somewhere between 5 and 10 percent of all those who enter the program. There is doubtless some portion of those people who would have gotten better on their own, as the data on spontaneous remission is impressive indeed. Still, it is clear that a small number of people get well in AA *because* of AA. How can we square this fact with all that I have discussed to this point, including the fact that AA's philosophy is deeply at odds with the psychology of addiction?

The voices of the addicts that we heard in the last chapter give us important clues. One of the principal benefits of AA is its social function. AA is a place where, with some notable exceptions, people feel accepted. Early in the process of quitting drinking, this can be valuable for those who can make use of it. But social support is not what AA identifies as its reason for success: the Twelve Steps are supposed to be the method for treating addiction. If AA's public statements or literature focused on the supportive benefits of the group and made no claims that it was a specific treatment for addiction, nobody would object. Likewise, rehabilitation centers based on AA would resolve most objections if they simply admitted that getting away from the stress of daily life and into a lovely setting with good food and friendly support was a major part of their effectiveness—and the primary reason their results don't last.

But support and setting alone cannot account for all of the cases where AA works to treat addiction. As we will see, there are some circumstances in which AA's approach matches an individual's psychology in something of a virtuous coincidence. Later in this chapter, I'll examine why AA works when it does, and try to make sense of this phenomenon through the prism of a more accurate model of addiction.

GROUP DYNAMICS

Time and again in AA's literature, we find the Twelve Steps referenced as the one true road map to lasting sobriety. You'll recall that the Big Book itself contains the sentence, "Rarely have we seen a person fail who has thoroughly followed our path."

But the scientific literature has had a harder time distilling AA's "secret sauce." Many studies, in fact, have found strong evidence that AA's successes are based on elements of the group that have *nothing at all* to do with the Twelve Steps. Because these factors are common to any group, anywhere, I will call them *general attributes.*

Much of the evidence about what AA actually does for people seems to point to the curative power of group dynamics more than any specific philosophy. This is hardly new ground in psychology: peer groups have been shown time and again to wield tremendous influence over our beliefs and behaviors, including several recent studies suggesting that similar effects may be witnessed in elementary school and even social networks such as Facebook.[1]

Many of the studies I have already mentioned cite the power of the group as essential to AA's action. Both McKellar and Kaskutas outlined these effects in some detail. Kaskutas notes: "Meetings provide an opportunity to share one's own struggles . . . increase one's motivation to abstain, and . . . get outside of one's self . . . by hearing others talk about their problems."[2] He also notes that other studies have found a link to factors such as developing a stronger friendship network. The Moos researchers made essentially the same point, stating that "for some individuals, involvement with a circle of abstinent friends may reflect a turning point that enables them to address their problems, build their coping skills, and establish more supportive social resources."[3] Even David Sack, AA apologist and CEO of the conglomerate that owns Promises Treatment Centers, says, "Health care professionals want to study treatment and that's understandable. But . . . AA's view is 'that's not our problem if you think it works or not because we are here to help and support each other.'"[4]

The common thread here is an ongoing tension between the idea of AA as a treatment, and the idea of AA as a "fellowship" whose power lies in a more general model of community. Most proponents of the program say that one cannot be teased apart from the other, that the fellowship (meetings) and the treatment (the Twelve Steps) create a harmonious whole that is greater than the sum of its parts. Yet the question remains: might *any* group of alcoholics or other drug addicts serve just as well as AA? Are the things that make AA unique—the Twelve Steps, the testimony, the sponsors, and so on—integral to its main action, or are they mostly an overlay that functions to create a structure for the organization, much like the rules and traditions common to other fraternal organizations?

One clue may lie in a piece advice that AA itself gives to new members. As Harris describes, AA "advocates that new members attend different groups until they find one that suits their needs."[5] If the Twelve Steps were a true treatment for addiction, should it matter whether one group is more suitable than another? The recommendation makes far more sense if we think of AA as a *fellowship rather than a treatment*. If the group *is* the point, then of course one would need to find the right group to experience the benefits.

THE QUESTION OF SPIRITUALITY

One of the pillars of AA often cited as central to its effectiveness is its strong emphasis on spirituality. The Twelve Steps are explicitly spiritual, and much has been made about the unique benefits of AA's notion of surrendering to a Higher Power. But the scientific literature is skeptical on this point. In his 2003 paper, Harris and colleagues looked specifically at the attitudes toward spirituality of people who had attended AA. What they found was illuminating:

> Roughly equal groups expressed "positive, "neutral" and "negative" current attitudes towards AA (38%, 36% and 26%, respectively). Each of these three AA-attitude groups expressed greater endorsement of "Personal Responsibility" steps than of "Higher Power mediated"

steps. . . . A clear and consistent pattern of endorsement was evident . . . with the majority agreeing with steps that do not explicitly mention God or a Higher Power but encourage acceptance, self-examination and reparation (grouped as "Personal Responsibility" steps). A considerable proportion reported the references to God (54.4%) and the Higher Power (62.4%) were "off-putting" (the term most commonly used in pilot interviews for adverse views).[6]

In other words, the steps that were explicitly spiritual or religious seemed to be more distasteful than useful, even among people who felt positive about their experiences in AA as a whole. In fact, the Harris study reported that "of patients with AA experience . . . [only] 2.8 percent had experienced a spiritual awakening." The authors added that "'Higher Power' endorsement was ($p < .001$) [very highly] predicted by [prior] religious involvement and lifetime number of AA meetings attended." In sum, people who came in religious stayed that way, but the majority did not seem to have been markedly affected by the ongoing emphasis on spiritual rebirth.

Another study, by J. Tonigan of the University of New Mexico, concluded that "[c]ontrary to AA doctrine, spirituality does not appear to exert a main effect on drinking reductions. . . . The path between spirituality and drinking reductions was non-significant."[7] A similar result was reported by Owen and colleagues (2003), who found that spirituality is "uniformly and regularly discussed in AA meetings . . . increased spiritual endorsement, however, was not predictive of increased abstinence."[8]

One of the interesting wrinkles in this discussion is the fact that AA famously disputes any notion that it's a religious organization at all. (Bill Wilson once said, without apparent irony, "Our Twelve Steps have no theological content, except that which speaks of 'God as we understand Him.' . . . There isn't the slightest interference with the religious views of any of our membership. The rest of the Twelve Steps define moral attitudes and helpful practices, all of them precisely Christian in character.")[9]

Our court system does not agree, however. According to the North Carolina School of Government, in court cases where people have been mandated to attend AA, "[W]hat's not at issue in these cases is the question of whether AA is, in fact, religion-based. The litigants typically agree that it is, and the courts are unpersuaded by the idea that it's 'spiritual' and not religious."[10] This fact has been echoed in more than ten court rulings across the United States, including this opinion by New York's Court of Appeals, the state's highest court:

> The foregoing demonstrates beyond peradventure that doctrinally and as actually practiced in the 12-step methodology, adherence to the A.A. fellowship entails engagement in religious activity and religious proselytization. Followers are urged to accept the existence of God as a Supreme Being, Creator, Father of Light and Spirit of the Universe. In "working" the 12 steps, participants become actively involved in seeking such a God through prayer, confessing wrongs and asking for removal of shortcomings. These expressions and practices constitute, as a matter of law, religious exercise for Establishment Clause purposes, no less than the nondenominational prayer in Engel v Vitale (370 US 421), that is, "a solemn avowal of divine faith and a supplication for the blessings of the Almighty. The nature of such a prayer has always been religious."[11]

That an organization judged by many unbiased parties to be religious would deny its religious orientation yet still point to those same religious principles as the key to its success, suggests confusion among its members about what makes AA work, and why.

Other theories about the possible therapeutic action of AA have been floated and discarded. A 2010 study of over seventeen hundred patients concluded, "The Alcoholics Anonymous (AA) literature states that reduction of anger is critical to recovery. . . . However, AA attendance was unrelated to changes in anger."[12] Tonigan and Rice noted that AA strongly encourages its members to develop a relationship with a sponsor. But their results showed that affiliation with a sponsor was unrelated to abstinence past the first months of joining.[13]

Why is it that no one can seem to isolate the specific things that make AA work for the people who find success in the program? As we will soon see, it is because questions of spirituality and group dynamics are ultimately beside the point. When AA works, it's due to other factors that are incidental to its main approach but dovetail with some elements of the psychology of addiction.

THE PSYCHOLOGY OF AA'S SUCCESS

You'll recall that I described addictive behavior as a response to feelings of overwhelming helplessness. It's what people do to "fight back" against this unbearable feeling. But addictive acts are never a direct way to fight back: they are substitutions (or displacements) for a direct action, taken precisely because taking a direct step is felt to be impossible or forbidden. One of the unique qualities of displacements is that they work in much the same way that the direct action might: for addicts, drinking a beer or placing a bet really *does* relieve the unbearable sensation that no options are available.

It's worth remembering as well that this searing, personal version of helplessness takes many forms and is wholly contingent on the psychology of the addict. I've seen patients whose most intolerable form of helplessness centers around a sense of abandonment, or being invisible, or feeling undistinguished professionally, or losing an argument. There are, in other words, as many addiction-driving forms of helplessness as there are addicts; no two are precisely the same. Our unique histories inform that which we find untenable.

Yet the number of substitute remedies for helplessness tends to be far lower. As we know, addiction is one of the most common. The causes may be diverse, but the function is always the same: to extinguish helplessness by replacing it with its opposite, empowerment. This fact—that addiction is ultimately a quest for empowerment—is the key to bridging the gap between what AA says and how AA really works. That key rests within the single term *higher power*.

Most of us start out life without a strong boundary between our individual selves and the world at large. Young children in particular tend to engage the world as a sort of composite "we"—part child, part parent. Numerous psychological studies have confirmed that children identify with their parents or caregivers far more when they're young than when they're older. And why shouldn't they? In this identification lies a great reservoir of comfort. When you align yourself with someone bigger and stronger than yourself, you can eliminate many of the scariest feelings of childhood—being weak, small, and unable to do most things. Identifying with a more powerful parent or caregiver is a healthy step in our emotional development, one that enables us to transition gracefully from infant to adult without spending every waking moment in a state of terror and confusion.

This same tendency to identify with powerful figures wends its way through our adulthood in certain ways. Witness the powerful identification many of us feel with great athletes, or entertainment stars, or even brands such as technology companies. (It's no coincidence that one of the most effective campaigns of the twenty-first century used the phrase, "I'm a Mac.") Studies have noted the very real sense in which the things that happen to our chosen heroes affect us as well, including a well-cited article that showed that men's testosterone levels tend to drop when their favorite sports team loses a big game.[14] The converse is true as well—we revel in our team's victories, own them as our own, and feel powerful for sharing the success.

In politics, too, our identities can rapidly become enmeshed with our favorite people and causes. Many leaders throughout history have depended on a similar psychology to powerfully influence their followers; Winston Churchill famously emboldened his people never to yield, and because they identified with his strength, his words proved to be a source of strength for them.

With this in mind, now let us return to the first three steps of Alcoholics Anonymous:

Step 1: "We admitted we were powerless over our addiction—that our lives had become unmanageable."

Step 2: "Came to believe that a Power greater than ourselves could restore us to sanity."

Step 3: "Made a decision to turn our will and our lives over to the care of God as we understood God."

It is hard to imagine a more explicit plea to engage in the same sort of psychology that adults feel with their heroes. What's interesting about these three steps is how differently addicts react to them. As we've seen, the majority of people in AA resist these ideas. These notions seem in a sense tailor-made to exacerbate the powerful sense of helplessness that most addicts are already struggling against.

But there is another possible response: some people, rather than pushing back against the "Higher Power" idea, accept it wholeheartedly. They do not perceive this notion as a threat to their autonomy, but as a great reservoir of power that they can draw upon. Since addiction is ultimately an effort to reverse helplessness, the idea that a benevolent and all-powerful entity is now on their side—in a sense, is a part of them—is deeply compelling. For those who can make use of this concept, it can be a genuine solution. As long as the Higher Power is seen as potent and reliable, a person who identifies with it may be able to abstain from addictive behavior; he or she no longer needs it to relieve helplessness.

But the primary concern about this method of achieving sobriety is its precarious quality. The relief afforded by the notion of a higher power is commensurate with the great disappointment one feels when that higher power turns out to be an illusion—or worse, an abusive force. This revelation is in a sense multiplied in its effect by the very scale of the power: the increase in confidence is great, and the betrayal can be just as devastating.

In 12-step programs, one of the most common ways the Higher Power can tumble is through a fault line in the sponsor-sponsee relationship. One of AA's founding principles is the notion that members who have achieved sobriety have useful wisdom and support to offer by virtue of their own success in holding off addiction. Alas, these people are typically as fallible as anyone else, and even long-standing members can lapse or even withdraw from the program. To sponsees—or "pigeons" in AA language—whose notion of the organization's power is intertwined with the sponsor's success story, events such as these can be devastating, leading to the return of addictive behavior.

Imagining AA itself as the Higher Power is equally problematic, since the organization can fail its members as well. Many addicts report bad experiences in groups they had hoped to rely upon, and the effects of these incidents can be far more damaging if they carry the meaning that the Higher Power has clay feet. Administrative slights, abusive members, and unwanted advances (a problem so common it's been given its own nickname: 13th stepping) can all poke holes in the idealized notion that many members cultivate around AA. To those whose sense of identity has become enmeshed with the group, exposing the man behind the curtain can be debilitating. At the very least, it leaves addicts who had relied on a Higher Power without emotional recourse.

If AA were more appropriately aware of how this mechanism works psychologically, it could make needed changes. But because AA's own theories about how it helps people are unsound, the organization tends to repeat the same problems in the same ways, disappointing and ultimately losing the vast majority of the people who try to benefit. Indeed, one of the most frustrating aspects of the program for many potential members is its repetitiveness in the face of clear contradictory evidence: AA members who lapse or struggle are prescribed nothing more or less than the original advice, perhaps delivered more loudly. Even those who can make use of AA as a remedy for helplessness are never taught or warned of the implicit dangers that come with this sort of powerful identification.

Another consequence of identifying strongly with an external Higher Power is that people are often left with little more understanding of themselves than when they began. The Twelve Steps strongly encourage members to seek power, solace, and strength from the group or from their notion of a High Power, but not from within themselves. (Some members do describe an increase in humility as a consequence of acknowledging their diagnosis and their step 4 "flaws," but greater humility is not relevant to the treatment of addiction.) Because no lasting psychological insights about addiction have been absorbed, gains made throughout sobriety can quickly evaporate as the addict discovers that the very same feelings of intolerable helplessness have returned, precisely as they were. For 12-step members who experience a Higher Power's fall from grace, as it were, the sensation can be like losing a limb—the thing they had leaned on for strength has vanished into thin air. People who grow to understand the psychology of addiction, on the other hand, are better prepared to deal with their addiction. Insight is a form of empowerment that cannot be wrested from your grasp.

One of the unfortunate consequences of AA's Higher Power success stories is the sensitivity that such a dependency foments. Since, for many of these people, sobriety depends on the integrity of what they believe, any challenge to those beliefs is felt to be a dangerous assault on the very thing that keeps them sober. The result is a well-documented tendency among AA members to aggressively defend the organization and its precepts without giving consideration to opposing ideas. Often AA skeptics and lapsed members find that current members respond with rage when pressed to consider different viewpoints or countermanding data. The visceral power of these responses should be a clue to the psychology behind them: we save our fiercest defenses for an attack on that which keeps us whole.

Speaking to professional groups around the country, I have regularly witnessed firsthand the energetic pushback AA members will typically deliver to anyone who dares to challenge AA dogma. Many times at these talks, I've been approached by therapists who tell me, often in a near-whisper, that they are deeply discouraged by the 12-step approach but are literally afraid to say anything for fear of losing their jobs. Their stories are awful, but the consequences are more so: if alternative views may not be uttered in these treatment centers, patients are prevented from hearing and thinking about them.

Because so many leaders and counselors within our nation's treatment programs are "recovering" addicts themselves, it can be tremendously difficult to begin a civil public conversation about the shortcomings of the approach, and more or less impossible to produce change in their treatment programs. The dominance of AA devotees in the addiction treatment industry extends as well to government agencies charged with providing services to addicts.

AA's views about how it works are largely based on foundational beliefs and fail to include any insight into what drives addiction or how AA disrupts or amplifies those drivers. One of the principal ways AA helps people is in its capacity as a community, where it supplies a number of general attributes that are universally present in any religious or fraternal group.

But there are some occasions when AA inadvertently meets an individual's need to feel powerful against helplessness, addressing the underlying psychology of addiction without intending to. AA's lack of insight, however, leaves it without any consistent capacity to correct its problems or expand its effectiveness. The same lack of awareness in those for whom AA "works," leads to a hostile incapacity to be thoughtful when presented with views that challenge their belief system.

What can be done to make use of that which is useful in the program? Since AA is helpful for a small minority of people with alcoholism, and often neutral or detrimental to others, it should be prescribed carefully. The current practice of referring addicts wholesale to a 12-step group is unwise and dangerous. In a rational system, every person with addiction would be individually evaluated with two questions:

Is the person capable of engaging in an introspective psychotherapy?

This question shouldn't be read as a prescription to go into psychoanalysis; it merely refers to the ability to be thoughtful about oneself and speak with a therapist about what is in one's heart and mind. Some of this work can be done on one's own by using the perspective on the psychology behind addiction, as I've described in other books. But to effectively root out the various unseen ways that we can become vulnerable to feeling overwhelmingly helpless, it is generally advisable to find a good therapist.

Is the person likely to make use of the 12-step approach?

People who make it clear they find 12-step meetings and ideas to be offensive, stupid, or wrong should not be encouraged to ignore their feelings. They are telling us in clear language that they are simply not candidates for this particular approach. Conversely, those who like 12-step programs and benefit from them are telling us they may belong in that small group of committed and helped members.

Directing people toward the best approach for them is one of the most basic forms of medical care. We have generally failed at applying thoughtful triage like this to addiction in this country. Twelve-step programs aren't appropriate for most, but there is no question that they can be helpful to the right sort of person. The better we are able to understand why and how this happens, the better we can provide more effective care across the board. That will mean ending the practice of routinely referring people to 12-step programs.

CHAPTER EIGHT

THE MYTHS OF AA

MYTHS HAVE A WAY of coming to resemble facts through repetition alone. This is as true in science and psychology as in politics and history. Today few areas of public health are more riven with unsubstantiated claims than the field of addiction.

Alcoholics Anonymous has been instrumental in the widespread adoption of many such myths. The organization's Twelve Steps, its expressions, and unique lexicon have found their way into the public discourse in a way that few other "brands" could ever match. So ingrained are these ideas, in fact, that many Americans would be hard-pressed to identify which came from AA and which from scientific investigation.

The unfortunate part of this cultural penetration is that many addiction myths are harmful or even destructive, perpetuating false ideas about who addicts are, what addiction is, and what is needed to quit for good. In this chapter, I'd like to take a look at a few of these myths and examine some of the ways they impair efforts at adopting a more effective approach.

MYTH #1: YOU HAVE TO "HIT BOTTOM" BEFORE YOU CAN GET WELL

This common myth essentially says that an addict needs to reach a point of absolute loss or despair before he or she can begin to climb back toward a safe and productive life.

The most common objection to this myth is simple logic: nobody can possibly know where their "bottom" is until they identify it in retrospect. One person's lowest point could be a night on the street, while another's could be a bad day at work or even a small personal humiliation. It's not unusual for one "bottom" to make way for another following a relapse. Without a clear definition, this is a concept that could be useful only in hindsight, if it is useful at all.

A bigger problem with this notion is the idea that addiction is in some fundamental way just a matter of stubbornness or stupidity— that is, addicts cannot recover until they are shown the consequences of their actions in a forceful enough way. This is a dressed-up version of the idea that addiction is a conscious choice and that stopping is a matter of recognizing the damage it causes. I have said it before, but it bears repeating: if consequences alone were enough to make someone stop repeating an addictive behavior, there would be no addicts. One of the defining agonies of addiction is that people can't stop despite being well aware of the devastating consequences. That millions of people who have lost their jobs, marriages, and families are still unable to quit should be a clear indication that loss and despair, even in overwhelming quantities, aren't enough to cure addiction. Conversely, many addicts stop their behavior at a point where they have not hit bottom in any sense.

There is a moralistic subtext at work here as well. The notion that addicts have to hit bottom suggests that they are too selfish to quit until they have paid a steep enough personal price. Once again we get an echo of the medieval notion of penance here: through suffering comes purity. Addicts no more need to experience devastating personal loss than does anyone else with a problem. Yes, it can be useful when a single moment helps to crystallize that one *has* a problem, but the fantasy that this moment must be especially painful is simply nonsensical.

Finally, the dogmatic insistence that addicts hit bottom is often used to excuse poor treatment. Treaters who are unable to help often scold addicts by telling them that they just aren't ready yet and that they should come back once they've hit bottom and become ready to do the work. This is little more than a convenient dodge for ineffectual care, and a needless burden to place on the shoulders of addicts.

MYTH #2: YOU MUST "SURRENDER" YOUR WILL TO GET WELL

Here we have another pillar of the Oxford Group, AA's theological forerunner, which preached salvation through surrender to God. In

Alcoholics Anonymous, this idea is implied, if not expressly stated, in steps 1 and 3, which respectively recommend admitting powerlessness and making a decision "to turn our will and our lives over to the care of God as we understood God."

The first problem with this idea is its overt religious flavor. I have covered the many ways that addiction is a problem of the mind and not of the spiritual soul. "Surrendering," in the sense that addiction organizations commonly understand it, means abdicating power to a presence greater than oneself to attain guidance. It's not surprising that many addicts chafe at this notion, not least because it requires a belief system that may not jibe with their own.

A bigger problem is that surrendering is tantamount to agreeing that one is incapable of managing one's own life. AA's literature ties this idea once again to a moralistic adage: "Our whole trouble had been the misuse of will power."[1] Surrendering becomes a way to toss out a useful sense of selfhood or agency precisely when it's needed most.

And of course the very notion of surrender is problematic when viewed through the prism of a more psychologically sophisticated understanding of addiction. As I outlined in chapter 5, the emotion that precipitates addiction is *helplessness*. Addicts find certain forms of helplessness utterly intolerable, and the addiction is an effort to reverse that. Asking them to surrender their free will in response to this problem is diametrically opposed to what they need to do: feel empowered. As we saw in the first-person accounts in chapter 6, the dissonance created by this emphasis on surrender is one of the big reasons so many addicts don't get better in AA.

MYTH #3: COUNTING YOUR DAYS
OF ABSTINENCE IS A USEFUL THING TO DO

Enter any conversation about AA with addicts "recovering" in AA, and they will likely be able to tell you the precise number of years, months, and days they've been sober. This is an integral part of Alcoholics Anonymous and its offshoots: a tally system designed to discourage backsliding by turning sobriety into something additive, an ever-expanding reward system. The AA tradition of giving out tokens or chips for days of sobriety is intended to be a helpful reminder of what people have accomplished, and a way to discourage them from falling off the wagon.

The dark side of this practice is what happens when addicts take a drink or slip in some way: they must go back to zero and lose everything they've gained. It's obvious that this system can cause a great deal of pain, and the humiliations that come with it can be manifold. Giving up tokens and esteem feels like—is *intended* to feel like—wiping out all the hard work that has come before and starting over. The moralistic dimension of this is hard to miss; some recovering addicts even use the tsk-tsk acronym SLIP (for *sobriety loses its priority*). If you are in AA and slip, you cannot avoid feeling like a failure, because that's exactly what the system is designed to tell you.

Yet slips are hardly rare and not remotely apocalyptic. Most people will experience some lapses as they grapple with their addiction. This is completely predictable, given the fact that addictions arise from deeply personal emotions and experiences that can take months and years to work through. To suggest that having a drink or placing a bet should "undo" all the progress an addict has made to date is absurd. That progress happened. And its benefits are no less cumulative for the interruption.

In fact, lapses can be turned into something useful, as I described in chapter 5. They can be a window into the personal nature of addiction that might guide addict and therapist toward a new understanding of what drives the behavior. If an addict's efforts at sobriety have been unbroken until a particular moment, then it is always worth digging into that moment in some detail to understand what precipitated the relapse. People with addictions often feel empowered by this ongoing process of investigation and liberated by the insights it yields.

MYTH #4: PEOPLE WITH ADDICTION ARE ALL THE SAME: "DRUNKS"

This language is AA's own, and lies at the heart of its one-size-fits-all treatment philosophy. In a sense, the word "drunks" is meant to be comforting, communal, a collective identity that defuses the terror of addiction and gives people a sense of belonging and a chance to laugh at their struggles. Unfortunately, the word is also reductive, and understandably disliked by many addicts. Its frequent use is designed to break down the barriers between group and self and to take down a peg those who come to meetings feeling that they don't really belong lumped in with everyone else. Individual identity of this sort is frowned upon in 12-step culture; "drunks" gives everyone the same deprecating title and the same implied prognosis for recovery.

It is not surprising that the word also serves the AA mission. Because this is a program where everybody receives the same treatment, it makes sense to call everyone by the same word. The word "drunks" also defines addicts by their addiction, further reinforcing the notion that addicts are somehow different from the rest of us, as if addiction is an innate quality rather than an acquired behavior. In the world of Alcoholics Anonymous, where alcoholics all supposedly suffer with the same character flaws and problems, addiction is not something you do, it's something you are.

The word thus ignores the tremendous variety of people who become addicts. Addiction appears within every possible socioeconomic level and in people who run the gamut of emotional health. To reduce this variety to just one word is to ignore the widely divergent experiences that can lead to addictive behavior. The core issues that lead to feelings of overwhelming helplessness, and thence to addiction, are as varied as the people who experience them. For some, this underlying distress may be about failing in competition; for others it may be about the loss of an important person, or an inability to protect themselves in a relationship. That all these people become "drunks" is almost beside the point. Their lives are what is significant. Using one word to describe them all shrugs off the individual treatment they require.

(A corollary to this label is the notion that people with addictions are pleasure-seekers: "Drunks" are people who can't keep themselves from the pleasure of getting drunk. But true addiction has almost nothing to do with a tendency to gorge on that which we find enjoyable; it persists long after the pleasure is gone.)

MYTH #5: "ONE DAY AT A TIME"

This famous slogan encapsulates the outside-in, behaviorally oriented nature of AA and its offshoots. AA members are constantly discouraged from thinking too far ahead, lest they become overwhelmed or disheartened. In a sense, this is an echo of the notion that addiction is innate—a steady and implacable force, not unlike gravity, that requires constant, effortful pushback. AA members do not speak of a cure because they view their addiction as fundamentally incomprehensible—not something to be understood and resolved, but something to be *resisted*. When addiction is seen this way, every day is more or less like every other day. Looking ahead offers no benefits.

The notion of taking things one day at a time is also rather infantilizing, as it suggests that addicts cannot bear the burden of considering weeks or months without addiction. This would make sense if abstinence were like lifting weights or running a marathon: it's useful to hang on to the "just one more" ethos to get through something that becomes increasingly difficult over time. But abstinence doesn't have to feel that way. A more appropriate metaphor would be learning a new instrument: you may start out one note at a time, but before long you are learning minuets and sonatas.

The biggest mistake with "One day at a time" is that it's backward. One of the truly useful things about understanding addiction from a psychological perspective is that this view breeds a kind of precognition: people become adept at predicting when the urge will arise.[2] In fact, thinking ahead is one of the most powerful tools in treatment, as it gives addicts a chance to head off their addictive urges long before those feelings actually occur. Purposely keeping one's head down and refusing to think about the future is a formula for getting blindsided by powerful and unfamiliar feelings.

MYTH #6: "STICK WITH THE WINNERS"

The idea that our behavior is influenced by our peer group is not unique to AA. The organization's exhortation to "stick with the winners" is a way of encouraging members to seek out positive role models in the program, but its unwanted consequences can be painful and isolating.

Speaking only with people who have "gotten sober" is a good way to miss out on hearing or learning from the great majority who do not find AA useful. AA members who attach themselves to successfully sober members may well discover that they cannot seem to reproduce the same results in the same way. This can quickly give way to shame, bitterness, and resignation. After all, these winners in AA typically will not thoughtfully evaluate newcomers to give the most fair-minded opinion of whether AA is best for them. And they especially won't advise anyone to look beyond AA for care.

There is a cruel dimension to this word choice as well: it strongly suggests that those who don't stick with AA are losers. As we have already seen, the vast majority of people who attend AA are more likely to "lose" than win. And addicts may well internalize this concept and consider it a mark of shame when their efforts do not produce lasting results, adding "loser" to their list of self-recriminations. And for the people who remain, the word "winners" comes with its own set of complications, including a tenuous sense of superiority that may suddenly be forfeited in the years ahead.

MYTH #7: "90 MEETINGS IN 90 DAYS"

Many new AA members are instructed to follow this slogan, which has informally arisen outside of AA's founding texts. Its purpose is to break the routine of addicts and get them instantly and deeply involved with the program and to help shake the destructive cycle they're in.

Alas, this particular prescription is essentially arbitrary. Like the thirty days almost universally recommended for rehabilitation centers, the ninety-day AA period is something pulled out of thin air, based on the intuition that three months should be enough time to get started on the right foot.

The 90/90 prescription, like other myths, has darker consequences as well. Even the most involved form of individual therapy—psychoanalysis (which I practice)—is almost always limited to four sessions a week. The idea that someone should make time for ninety consecutive days of meetings or risk feeling like a failure strains credulity. This is especially difficult for people who retain close relationships to friends or family, for whom being away from home frequently may stress already strained bonds.

The concept of "90 meetings in 90 days" sets people up for failure. Of course there are no actual consequences for missing a day, but the sense of obligation is real and carries its own emotional burden. Greeting someone just starting to address an addiction with such an arduous task is poor planning indeed.

MYTH #8: PEOPLE WITH ADDICTIONS HAVE CHARACTER DEFECTS

This idea is embedded in step 6—"*Were entirely ready to have God remove all these defects of character*"—and over time, it has been expanded in subsequent AA thought and literature. Here is one list of potential defects in addicts from an AA pamphlet:

1. Resentment, Anger
2. Fear, Cowardice
3. Self pity
4. Self justification
5. Self importance, Egotism
6. Self condemnation, Guilt
7. Lying, Evasiveness, Dishonesty
8. Impatience
9. Hate
10. False pride, Phoniness, Denial
11. Jealousy
12. Envy
13. Laziness
14. Procrastination
15. Insincerity
16. Negative Thinking
17. Immoral thinking
18. Perfectionism, Intolerance
19. Criticizing, Loose Talk, Gossip
20. Greed[3]

The idea that addicts have character defects is demonstrably false unless one includes in the definition of "character defects" all that makes us human. One problem with this idea is its universalizing nature: to suggest that all addicts suffer from the same defects of character is to strongly imply that all addicts are the same, or close enough. This notion is consonant with the AA philosophy, but fails to comport with real-world evidence. There are addicts who are lazy and addicts who are driven; greedy alcoholics and alcoholics who are selfless to a fault. Notably, these attributes cannot be demonstrated to be any more common in addicts than anyone else.

In terms of treatment, admitting that one suffers from these character defects is also irrelevant. Of course, the goal of treatment is to understand oneself better, and a candid self-evaluation comes with the territory. But the suggestion that one could ever cure an addiction by trying to be less critical of people, or by gossiping less, or by trying to think positively, is nonsensical. And the implicit message that addicts must catalog their flaws to get better is disrespectful.

What's really behind the "character defects" myth is the old idea that to beat addiction, you should try to be a better person. From there it's a short leap to the inference that addicts are bad people. This notion wends its way through the Big Book in any number of places, and reaches back through time to the Oxford Group and its foundational emphasis on sinning and salvation. It is a moralistic approach designed to engender contrition, compel surrender, and ultimately to rebuild people as better citizens. But it has nothing to do with addiction.

MYTH #9: ONLY AN ADDICT CAN TREAT AN ADDICT

This has been one of the most widely believed of AA's myths and one that continues to do harm. The assumptions behind it are twofold: (1) only an addict can understand and relate to the experience of addiction, and (2) the only counselor an addict will trust is someone who has been through that experience.

To the extent that any part of this myth has merit, it lies in the second assumption. It may be hard for some people with addictions to place their trust in the hands of someone who has not experienced addiction. This usually has to do with the shame an addict may bring to the therapy: *If I feel so terrible about myself, you must feel the same way about me, unless you have the same problem.* Of course, personally having an addiction is irrelevant to the ability of therapists, and part of any good therapy is working through mistrustful feelings together and ultimately developing a lasting trust based on compassion, insight, and a shared goal.

But the first assumption is fundamentally wrong: there is no truth to the notion that one must be an addict to treat an addict. Since addiction is a psychological phenomenon, it stands to reason that the best person to treat an addict would be someone who has trained in psychology. Of course that person might *also* be an addict, but his or her personal experience is essentially irrelevant. To elevate a personal history of addiction into a credential on its own is to miss out on the manifold benefits of professional training.

The idea that only an addict can treat an addict has led to the rise of thousands of "addiction counselors" whose only credential is their status as recovering addicts. At minimum, this treatment community does a disservice to addicts by practicing therapy without formal education; at worst, some of these recovering addicts may be seriously unfit to perform this work. A common consequence is counselors who simply repeat the Twelve Steps and recommend whatever worked for them, then express bewilderment and frustration when it doesn't work for their patients.

This philosophy appears in the sponsorship model as well, which relies heavily on the notion that someone who has remained abstinent must possess useful wisdom that a newer member can use. But sponsors regularly impart their personal experience, not wisdom gathered from knowledge or a deeper understanding of the problem. And sponsors may eventually succumb to relapse, which is something few professional therapists have to worry about.

In the end, the myth that only an addict can treat an addict is also an insult. The idea that having an addiction makes people so different from others that only other addicts could possibly understand them is demeaning. Nobody would ever suggest that a doctor must have had cancer to treat cancer, yet in the 12-step model, addiction is accorded this special designation of "otherness."

MYTH #10: "THE DEFINITION OF INSANITY IS DOING THE SAME THING OVER AND OVER AND EXPECTING A DIFFERENT RESULT"

This homily (often apocryphally attributed to Albert Einstein) has found its way into popular culture, but it claims a special place in AA, whose members use it as a cudgel against themselves and each other for drinking when they should know better. Those of us who work in clinical psychiatry could tell you that this isn't remotely close to the definition of insanity. Doing the same thing over and over again and expecting a different result is, at worst, a symptom of self-deception, or perhaps unfounded hope.

More to the point, addiction itself isn't a remotely insane thing to do. Addiction has its own logic and its own purpose, as we've seen. And although addicts may engage in deeply destructive behavior, crazy they are not. People with addictions are usually quite aware of the reality and consequences of what they're doing, including the painful knowledge that it "makes no sense." They might *feel* crazy, but once an addict understands the psychology behind his or her behavior, that feeling often gives way to a more empowering sense of personal insight.

Like so many of the other myths detailed in this chapter, the insanity myth is too often used as a way to diminish addicts and to scold them for their behavior. Like the other AA credos we have examined, this one implies that addiction is a purely conscious choice, that willpower (or turning your will over to an omnipotent Higher Power) is all you need to quit, and that recognizing the irrationality of your behavior should be enough to jar you out of your addictive haze.

MYTH #11: "DENIAL AIN'T JUST A RIVER IN EGYPT"

This expression wasn't coined by AA, but it has been adopted by the recovery community. AA's literature often mentions denial as one of the key personal defects that lets addicts persist in their behavior. (The fourth edition of the Big Book even has a section called "Crossing the River of Denial," which begins, "Denial is the most cunning, baffling and powerful part of my disease, the disease of alcoholism.") It isn't hard to imagine where this myth came from. It's based on a genuine phenomenon, namely that people with addictions often deny that, in fact, they have an addiction. But this denial is less about a failure to recognize reality than a natural need to reject the label "addict" and all the baggage that comes with it.

Recall that reversing helplessness is a core element in the psychology of addiction. Asking an addict to admit that he has an addiction understandably creates strong resistance, because it feels to him like being asked to admit helplessness itself. But when people understand how addiction works psychologically—as a fundamentally healthy drive to feel empowered when it seems like there is no other choice, I have often seen their denial melt away. It turns out that AA's emphasis on denial is misplaced; denial itself isn't the problem—it's shame, coupled with a lack of understanding of the nature of addiction that makes "denial" necessary.

The denial myth is yet another way that addicts and their loved ones infantilize and insult those who suffer from addiction. It fits all too well with the narrative of addiction as a form of "insanity" performed by people with "character defects," whose experience is so alien than only a fellow addict can ever save them. These ideas are understandable expressions of frustration recorded by people who look at the seeming illogic of addiction and throw up their hands in exasperation. But they do terrible harm to the very addicts whose recovery depends on understanding themselves without judgment.

Addiction seems to hold a special place in the American imagination. It is categorized as somehow different and separate from the problems and symptoms we all suffer. Partly as a result of this singular and mysterious strangeness, addiction is treated less like a common psychological symptom and more like a cultural one. In the absence of sophisticated knowledge, platitudes and homilies rush in to fill the void, many of which obscure far more than they illuminate. Folklore and anecdote are elevated to equal standing with data and evidence. Everyone's an expert, because everyone knows somebody who has been through it. And nothing in this world travels faster than a pithy turn of phrase.

CHAPTER NINE

THE FAILURE OF ADDICTION RESEARCH AND DESIGNING THE PERFECT STUDY

ONE OF THE MOST galling aspects of the current approach to addiction treatment is how little research is being done to seek better solutions. Despite all the failings of research on 12-step effectiveness, the field has come to a consensus around the idea that 12-step programs are useful and have been sufficiently studied. A review of the most recent three years (2010–2012) of the *American Journal on Addictions* shows no articles on or about 12-step programs. Two articles about 12-step treatment were published over the same period in the *Journal of Substance Abuse Treatment*, but neither examined either the effectiveness or mechanism of action of AA. There are, however, a number of papers whose purpose is simply to support 12-step treatment; Christine Timko, for example, published an article in the *Journal of Drug and Alcohol Dependence* with the stated goal of implementing and evaluating procedures "to help clinicians make effective referrals to 12-step self-help groups."[1]

Addiction research has for years followed the prevailing trade winds in popular science, folding itself into ever smaller cul-de-sacs of genetics and biochemistry. Studies of this kind are easy to fund (because they suggest pharmacological solutions supplied by drug manufacturers) and widely cited, helping to perpetuate the illusion that someday advances in molecular science might reduce complex human behavior to the ingredients in a few synaptic cocktails.

Alas, these approaches are doomed by their reductive scope and hampered by an issue of expertise. The research is inevitably conducted by biologists who have little or no training in the psychology of human addiction. This is not to say they aren't competent scientists. We become experts in the things we do; these researchers are without question the world's foremost experts on the study of rat brains. But to apply a rat-based dopamine study to a deeply intricate problem like human addiction is to neglect the wealth of knowledge and experience we have gained from treating humans.

The big problem that underlies such half-a-loaf takes on addiction is the absence of psychological awareness in the major addiction journals. This neglect is no accident: views not fitting with the present biochemical paradigm are simply not accepted for publication. (I have witnessed this firsthand as both a reviewer and an author.) What passes for psychological insight in the professional addiction literature are virtually always simple questionnaires that rank people according to superficial traits such as "interest in risky activities." This absence of sophistication makes it impossible for these journals to recognize or meaningfully engage the psychology behind addictive behavior; there is simply no room for that conversation.

The other seismic shift in scientific literature that has strangled attempts to treat addiction from a psychological perspective is the injection of numbers into anything and everything that will harbor them. Most people who do good work in education or the humanities know that deeply significant truths cannot be measured. Great teaching, for example, is hard to quantify. Most good, worthy, and verifiable ideas don't belong in a spreadsheet. Yet as a result of insecurity or ignorance, the majority of scientific publications today won't even consider a paper that isn't larded with numbers from top to bottom.

The consequence of this institutional blindness to qualitative and nuanced thought is that research is typically limited to broad statistical studies that do not investigate causes or meanings. In addiction research, these large population survey studies never once ask any questions about the feelings inside the people they are examining. As a consequence, they are often astonishingly obvious or trivial. Here are just a few recent examples from the major addiction journals:

"How Do Prescription Opioid Users Differ From Users of Heroin or Other Drugs in Psychopathology?" (*Journal of Addiction Medicine*)

> This article statistically analyzed over nine thousand survey records (no people were interviewed), concluding the painfully obvious fact that using drugs such as heroin and morphine is correlated with the likelihood of using other drugs, being depressed and anxious, and having a lower "quality of life."[2]

"Health/Functioning Characteristics, Gambling Behaviors, and Gambling-Related Motivations in Adolescents Stratified by Gambling Problem Severity: Findings from a High School Survey" (*American Journal on Addictions*)

> This article statistically analyzed data from a survey of over twenty-four hundred high school students. Its conclusion was that pathological gambling was associated with poor academic performance, depression, and aggression. The authors said their findings suggested a need for better interventions with adolescents who gamble.[3]

"What Is Recovery? A Working Definition from the Betty Ford Institute" (*Journal of Substance Abuse Treatment*)

> This article states that it fills the (presumed) need for a standard definition of the word *recovery*. It solves this problem as follows: "Recovery is a voluntarily maintained lifestyle characterized by sobriety, personal health, and citizenship." Incredibly, this paper is listed as among the five "most cited" references for the entire *Journal of Substance Abuse Treatment*.[4]

"Effect of Alcohol References in Music on Alcohol Consumption in Public Drinking Places" (*American Journal on Addictions*)

> This paper describes a study designed to test "whether textual references to alcohol in music played in bars lead to higher revenues of alcoholic beverages." The results were that "customers who were exposed to music with textual references to alcohol spent significantly more on alcoholic drinks." Mind you, this article didn't appear in a hospitality

trade publication presumably because marketing people could have told you this already.[5]

"Psychosocial Stress and Its Relationship to Gambling Urges in Individuals with Pathological Gambling" (*American Journal on Addictions*)

The title of this paper gives promise that the study will employ some psychological sophistication. Alas, its conclusion puts such hopes to rest: "Patients with PG [pathological, or compulsive, gambling] displayed significantly higher scores on the daily stress inventory . . . than did healthy subjects. These findings support the role of psychosocial stress in the course of PG."[6] There is no mention of how this stress functions, why it drives addiction, or any aspect of human psychology that might help to explain and deepen the paper's obvious conclusion.

What's missing from this literature is any study that revisits the fundamental questions once and for all: What is addiction? How should we treat it? Why does it occur in some individuals and not others?

I mentioned earlier that in the 1990s, one attempt at such a study was conducted by the National Institute on Alcohol Abuse and Alcoholism. But the study, called "Project MATCH," was severely limited in many ways. Most significantly, it looked at only three approaches: cognitive behavior therapy, "motivational enhancement" therapy, and 12-step treatment. It concluded that no difference in outcomes could be found among these. There was no control group and no psychodynamic group. Given the study's design, it is not surprising that the results were so disappointing, and that serious questions have been raised about whether any of these treatments were effective at all.[7]

What would it take to answer the question of how we should treat addiction? A definitive addiction study could potentially be designed, funded, and executed. A study of this kind would provide a blueprint for research panels at the NIH and universities and give lay readers a far better way to interpret the headlines that constantly trumpet yet another breakthrough about addiction. Most importantly, a truly meaningful study would be long enough to measure true growth and change, versus the prevailing short-term glances at transient benefits. Before discussing how such a study could be created, I must first address some key issues that have interfered with proper acceptance of serious psychological research in the addiction literature.

THE MIRAGE OF "EVIDENCE-BASED" SCIENCE

One of the impediments to including psychological understanding in addiction research is the wildly popular idea that only "evidence-based" treatment is worthwhile. It is useful to examine whether this idea has merit.

Most people with a scientific bent would agree that science is based on evidence. Without strong supporting corroboration, we would have no way to distinguish between a gut feeling and a solid result, and no way to separate personal bias from objective fact. But the value of evidence depends entirely on whether the data is meaningful—whether it is valid (bears on the topic) and important. No field, from the hardest statistical science to the "softest" sociology, is immune to abuses of the word "evidence"; some just do a better job of hiding their foundational biases than others. As we have seen, the use of "evidence" in addiction studies is no guarantee that the numbers will be treated without bias or even that they represent anything useful. As we have also seen, the majority of addiction studies covering 12-step treatment fail to pass basic threshold standards of experimental control and causal inference. Yet these flawed methodologies are not always apparent to the lay reviewer, and the press hardly helps matters with its ongoing confusion between controlled science and meaningless correlations. As a consequence, much of what we are sold under the billing of evidence is simply *data*. And data without context is *noise*.

Consider just a few of the problems in widely cited articles on addiction (noted in chapter 5): compliance bias, lack of controls, inadequate length of study, ignoring data that would interfere with the study's conclusions (dropout data, for instance), statistically dubious extrapolations, logically unfounded leaps from rats to people, and a number of advanced statistical regression methods designed to retroactively account for all of these (though these methods have had only mixed success—biostatisticians would be the first to admit that even the most sophisticated tricks of the field cannot "fix" a study that isn't designed thoughtfully from the beginning).

And there is an even greater problem with the worship of evidence, regardless of its validity: it is very easy to find meaningless evidence. Setting up an experiment to study an irrelevant question is a bit like a telescope pointing at the wrong place—you may confirm that the sun is indeed hot, but if you're looking for life on Mars, then you haven't exactly advanced the dialogue. Experiments that are designed to answer facile or specious questions about their topics are doomed to irrelevance before they begin. Thus we have a parade of statisticians determined to figure out how many heroin addicts are likely to use cocaine, without bothering to ask if this data is actionable or illuminating. It can easily be "proven" that environmental cues remind us to drink or that compulsive gamblers tend to do poorly in school. You could send out a survey tomorrow and collect solid evidence that drinkers like to smoke or that there is more alcohol consumption when people are "stressed." You might even publish and advance in academia for having done so, while just out of sight, the state of addiction research remains in stasis.

Nearly every addiction study is guilty of looking at the wrong things, and the reason is that most of these researchers have no training or interest in psychology. The false dogma that addiction is a biochemical disorder, or can be understood with superficial measures of behavior, has become self-perpetuating in the addiction literature. The gatekeepers who stand at the threshold of our science journals continue to reward trivial inquiries that shore up this woefully inadequate model of human behavior. If more researchers considered psychological explanations of addiction—and they should, given the preponderance of countervailing evidence that has left the "brain disease" concept in tatters (remember the veterans' study discussed in chapter 5)—they might take an interest in more humanistic ideas about humans.

If someone wanted to study the psychology of addiction statistically (more on why this is not a great idea later), researchers could step away from the rats and examine what precipitates addictive actions in humans. In my second book, I raised this notion as a way to help people predict the next episode of addictive behavior.[8] The same question could be studied in a large-scale way by asking people to keep a record of the events, feelings, and situations that precede addictive acts. Subjects could then be interviewed to see if a common emotional thread can be found behind each of these precipitants. We might gather a good amount of evidence and find statistically significant commonalities in that data, suggesting that addiction is a comprehensible psychological symptom. No one has yet tried.

There is one other serious problem with the term "evidence-based science," and it was highlighted eloquently in a now-famous paper by John Ioannidis, a professor of medicine and director of the Stanford Prevention Research Center at Stanford University School of Medicine.[9] Ioannidis showed that a research finding is less likely to be true when the studies conducted in a field are smaller, when effect sizes are smaller (the difference between a positive and negative finding is small), when researchers are prejudiced in favor of or against a certain result, and perhaps most importantly, when studies make fundamentally inaccurate assumptions about whether their findings will be true before they run the study (more on this below). I have seen all of these errors in addiction research: an inadequate number of people in studies, attempts to find statistical meaning in a small effect (an overall success rate of 12-step treatment of only 5 to 10 percent), and bias in presenting data (selection bias, compliance bias, omitting data that doesn't fit the conclusion).

The error of starting out with the belief that what you are looking for is likely to be meaningful was first formally recognized by Thomas Bayes, an eighteenth-century English minister and mathematician. He wrote that in experimental science, it is necessary to estimate the chance of each result *prior* to running an experiment. A good example of why this is important was given by the statistician Nate Silver (famous for accurately predicting virtually every state and national election result in the United States in both 2008 and 2012).[10] Silver points out how, for many years, the winner of the Super Bowl was widely said to predict the rise or fall of the stock market for the rest of that year. This was because starting with the first Super Bowl in 1967 and for the next thirty years until 1997, the stock market gained an average of 14 percent for the rest of the year when a team from the original NFL won the game, but fell almost 10 percent when a team from the original AFL won. Statistically, that correlation "showed" a definite connection between the two events. Indeed, there was just a one in five million possibility that this connection was due to chance alone! Without a foundation in Bayesian thinking, one would believe this to be incontrovertible proof that some as-yet-unidentified factor really did tie these two outcomes together. Of course they were mistaken, as the next fourteen years showed exactly the opposite result.

Bayes was intrigued by our tendency to seize upon absurd statistical conclusions like this and realized that relying on numbers alone was simply too shortsighted to make sense of statistics, or the world. Numbers contain precious little information about whether a correlation actually reflects a plausible reality or might instead be a statistical blip, hiccup, clump, or random anomaly.

In the case of the Super Bowl, for instance, those who breathlessly repeated and studied the coincidence as if it were significant forgot to ask an important question in plain language first: How could the winner of the Super Bowl have anything to do with the stock market? Bayes said that if you don't take into account the likelihood of something being true *before* you interpret the results, then you are stepping into never-never land; failing to decide in advance whether the outcome is realistic robs us of any chance to describe reality. For the Super Bowl correlation, a moment's thought would have given the likelihood of it being meaningful a very low probability. Applying Bayes' theorem (a simple formula that takes into account the likelihood of an outcome's being meaningful) would have yielded a result showing a very low chance that this measured statistic had any validity for the real world. As Ioannidis put it: "The probability that a research finding is indeed true depends on the prior probability of it being true (before doing the study), the statistical power of the study, and the level of statistical significance."[11]

All the studies we have seen purporting to show the effectiveness of AA, for instance, begin with the assumption that the AA method is eminently reasonable. As proof, they offer references to each other. In investigating these papers, I found zero references to psychological views of addiction, which might have led the authors to decrease their estimate of the likelihood that their results were describing anything of value. In an insular field that has preemptively decided what it believes, meaningless findings are reinforced and consonant results are amplified without the counterbalance of skepticism. Ioannidis said it best:

> The greater the . . . interests and prejudices in a scientific field, the less likely the research findings are to be true. Conflicts of interest and prejudice may increase bias [and] are very common in biomedical research, and typically they are inadequately and sparsely reported. . . . Scientists in a given field may be prejudiced purely because of their belief in a scientific theory or commitment to their own findings. . . . Prestigious investigators may suppress via the peer review process the appearance and dissemination of findings that refute their findings, thus condemning their field to perpetuate false dogma. . . . Empirical evidence on expert opinion shows that it is extremely unreliable.[12]

The root of this error goes beyond mutually supporting belief systems. The addiction field has been dominated by two colossal institutions, neither of which is trained or interested in looking beneath the surface of any behavior to its underlying causes. One of these forces is AA. The other is the titanic shift in psychiatry away from the exploration of human psychology toward more reductive and behavioral models, including the very popular notion that addiction is a disease. Both are riddled with biases that preclude their investigation of more plausible mechanisms behind addiction.

The end goal of those who study human behavior for genetic markers and neurotransmitters is a seductive fallacy: the notion that someday, with perfect knowledge of our brain chemistry, we might somehow "unlock" the essence of human experience. It is a fallacy because it fails to recognize what more than thirty years of chaos and complex systems theory have already taught us: When networked pieces of *anything* come together, be they ants in a colony or neurons in a brain, the network exhibits *emergent* behaviors that are far more strange and complex than anyone could predict from looking at their constituent parts. Indeed, one of the tantalizing findings of this research is that often these behaviors have *nothing to do* with those constituent parts; they are, in a sense, *platform agnostic*. One of my favorite quotes by the Nobel laureate Philip Anderson encapsulates the point wonderfully: "Psychology is not applied biology, nor is biology applied chemistry."[13]

How do I know that my own bias toward a psychological perspective isn't pushing me toward the same flawed and unfounded worldview? First, there is the commonsense fact that addiction looks just like known psychologically caused compulsions and can respond to purely psychological treatment; from a Bayesian standpoint, the idea that addictions and compulsions are intimately related is a sensible hypothesis. Those in favor of a biochemical model must contend with the fact that behaviors that truly are biochemical in origin, such as schizophrenia and mania, are fundamentally different from human addiction— they can arise and persist without psychological precipitants and can be treated with medication. Although these biochemical diseases create enormous distress, they do not have a specific emotional meaning or purpose; when appropriately treated with medication, people with these diagnoses can return to their usual state.

There are other objective factors supporting a psychological view of addiction. As we know from a large academic literature (see *The Heart of Addiction* for many references), as well as from common experience, addiction in humans follows psychological precipitants, which are idiosyncratic to each individual and predictable.[14] Addictive behavior can shift to compulsive symptoms that are universally understood to be psychological in nature, such as compulsively cleaning the house. And addiction can be successfully understood and treated by understanding how it works psychologically in each person through a talking treatment (psychotherapy). If we had never started out with the misconception that addictions are somehow different from other compulsive symptoms, we would not have made the error of separating them from the rest of the human condition to begin with.

WHEN NUMBERS MEAN LESS THAN WORDS

These days, virtually every addiction journal assigns far more value to statistical studies than to clinical findings. The primary claim is that words are not rigorous; numbers are. Yet this perspective fails to account for the complexity of human beings, who are, let's face it, not just more complex than rats, but more complex than any number could possibly assimilate. (If someone undergoes therapy and is now more comfortable in intimate situations, what number should we assign to that?)

Serious psychology journals usually manage this problem by reporting case studies rather than numbers. While individual cases have the limitation that they may not be generalizable to everyone, the accumulated wisdom from many case reports allows increased understanding of the way human beings' minds work. If you wanted to learn about how radios work, you could take a thousand of them and subject them to an experiment, say, by dropping them off a building, then study the statistical likelihood of their having transistors. Or, you could start with one radio and carefully take it apart. True, there might be other radios that work differently, but after examining this one, you would know in broad strokes how radios work.

Case reports have tremendous value. They are, quite simply, the only way to describe treatment. They supply a level of detail, nuance, and narrative that doesn't conform to statistical terms but contains more information. Therapy often yields common external and observable consequences of internal changes, but these may be impossible to measure except in the subjective experience of the patient. In the case of increased ability to tolerate intimacy, for instance, if a patient who has avoided closeness his entire life is now able to look someone in the eye and spend time talking instead of quickly hurrying away, that may be evidence of a life-changing alteration of his internal state that is deeply meaningful to the patient—yet ultimately immeasurable. Should we therefore discount it? Someone once said, "Not everything that is important can be measured, and not everything that can be measured is important." This is nowhere more applicable than in the study of human emotions, behaviors, and experience. We don't have a system of numbers for such things. But they couldn't be more relevant to the question of addiction.

The memorable phrase "Lies, damn lies, and statistics," commonly attributed to Mark Twain, was probably invented out of a combination of humor and pique. But statistics are neither good nor bad. In this book, I have cited statistics when there is no reason to doubt their legitimacy and criticized them when they are applied with bias or other methodological flaws. Perhaps most important, there are places where statistics have no role.

DESIGNING THE PERFECT STUDY

So how could we arrive at a more encompassing and broadly applicable consensus about what "works" in addiction treatment? The gold standard in science is the randomized controlled study. (No psychological study can be double-blind, which is the third common standard, as the psychologists administering the therapy will know which type of treatment they are offering.)

Let's imagine what that study might look like. A large population (over multiple treatment centers around the country) would be randomly assigned into groups that would receive the standard of care in four different approaches, or modalities: cognitive behavioral therapy (CBT), psychodynamic therapy based on the modern understanding described in this book, a 12-step outpatient approach, and a control group given no treatment at all. All groups would be matched for relevant factors such as age, sex, race, income, and educational levels. Follow-up surveys and interviews would be conducted every month through the six-month mark, and then at one year, two years, three years, five years, ten years, and twenty years.

Shockingly, nobody has ever conducted such a study. Besides a dismaying lack of interest, the other reason is almost certainly money. Major public studies such as these can run well into the millions of dollars.

And the organizations with the deepest pockets in this area have the strongest reasons to leave the current paradigm alone. It must ultimately fall to public science or to a wealthy university to get this kind of research off the ground. A fraction of what Americans spend on rehab would cover the entire study, and then some.

But the researchers would face some profound limitations as well. Psychodynamic work requires long-term follow-up, as well as assessment of outcomes beyond the symptom. One reason psychodynamic work requires long follow-ups is that major life-affecting improvement may occur during the treatment but before the addictive behavior ends. Therefore if the behavior alone is measured, then psychodynamic therapy may appear to be slower (hence less "effective") when what is actually happening is that the causes of the behavior are being worked out before the behavior stops (though the addiction may end before the therapy is very far along, as I described in *Breaking Addiction*).

The relative capacity of therapists would also have to be determined, which is much harder to do than establishing baseline competence to administer questionnaires or perform therapy out of a workbook (commonplace for CBT). However, no universal standard of effectiveness for psychodynamic work has ever been established. In order to adequately test the theory of addiction I've described in my work, it would be necessary to train already-sophisticated psychodynamic clinicians in this new perspective. The good news is that this would actually not be difficult, since the model is entirely based on already established and accepted psychodynamic understandings.

The costs and logistics of doing a proper study would certainly be great, but could be completed with governmental support. Unfortunately, the government's own agency (the National Institute on Drug Addiction) is deeply invested in its own neurobiological ("brain disease") idea. And pharmaceutical companies, a ready source for research on drugs, would have nothing to gain by funding a study of psychodynamic treatment.

For the time being, until a critical mass is reached on pursuing the question of addiction treatment from a fuller perspective, the very best contribution individuals can make is to seek out therapists with good general psychological training (and without 12-step bias), and to apply pressure where it is needed to mount a public campaign in support of enlightenment in addiction research.

My hope is that the website for this book will become a rallying point for readers to coalesce around the disillusionment so many Americans feel with the current system—and provide a tipping point that leads us toward a better approach to this solvable problem.

ACKNOWLEDGMENTS

WE ARE DEEPLY GRATEFUL to have had Helene Atwan as our editor. Her careful attention and perceptive eye made the book as good as it could be.

We would like to thank our agent, Don Fehr of Trident Media Group, whose enthusiasm for producing a potentially controversial book was essential to its creation.

Thanks also to Professor Richard Gelber, whose expertise in biostatistics was critical to our evaluation of scientific studies.

We are grateful to the many people who offered to share, by interview or in writing, their personal experiences with AA and rehab centers.

Lance would also like to thank the people he has seen in treatment over the years who have shared their experiences with addictions and the inner stories of their lives.

NOTES

CHAPTER ONE

1. Benedict Carey, "Drug Rehabilitation or Revolving Door?," *New York Times*, December 22, 2008.
2. L. Amato Ferri and M. Davoli: "Although it is the most common, AA is not the only 12-step intervention available. There are other 12-step approaches (labeled Twelve Step Facilitation (TSF). . . . No experimental studies unequivocally demonstrated the effectiveness of AA or TSF approaches for reducing alcohol dependence or problems" ("Alcoholics Anonymous and Other 12-Step Programmes for Alcohol Dependence," *Cochrane Database Systems Review* 3 [July 2006]: CD005032).
3. *Alcoholics Anonymous*, 3rd ed. (New York: AA World Services, 1976), 58–60.
4. Ibid., 77.
5. Paul Pringle, "The Trouble with Rehab, Malibu-Style," *Los Angeles Times*, October 9, 2007.

CHAPTER TWO

1. W. White, *Slaying the Dragon: The History of Addiction Treatment and Recovery in America* (Bloomington, IL: Chestnut Health Systems, 1998).
2. *Selected Papers of William L. White* website, "Significant Events in the History of Addiction Treatment and Recovery in America," http://www.williamwhitepapers.com/.
3. Cynthia Crossen, "If Dr. Keeley Could See You Now," *Wall Street Journal*, December 31, 2007.
4. Ibid.
5. M. Keller, "The Old and the New in the Treatment of Alcoholism," in *Alcohol Interventions: Historical and Sociocultural Approaches* (supplement to *Alcoholism Treatment Quarterly*), ed. B. Carruth et al. (New York: Routledge, 1986).
6. M. S. Gold, MD, and Christine Adamec, *The Encyclopedia of Alcoholism and Alcohol Abuse* (New York: Facts on File, 2010).
7. *Selected Papers of William L. White*, "Significant Events in the History of Addiction Treatment and Recovery."
8. B. Weiner and W. White, "The Journal of Inebriety (1876–1914): History, Topical Analysis, and Photographic Images," *Addiction* 102, no. 1 (January 2007): 15–23.

9. Francis Hartigan, *Bill W.: A Biography of Alcoholics Anonymous Cofounder Bill Wilson* (New York: St. Martin's Griffin, 2001). Unless otherwise indicated, in this chapter, quotes from and anecdotes about Bill Wilson are taken from this book.

10. William James, *The Varieties of Religious Experience* (CreateSpace Independent Publishing Platform, March 11, 2013).

11. *"Pass It On": The Story of Bill Wilson and How the A. A. Message Reached the World*, 1st ed. (New York: AA World Services, December 1984); also "Bill W.," *Wikipedia*, http://en.wikipedia.org/wiki/Bill_W.#cite_note-19.

12. B. Pittman, *AA: The Way It Began* (Seattle: Glen Abbey Books, 1988).

13. *"Pass It On."*

14. Susan Cheever, *My Name Is Bill: Bill Wilson—His Life and the Creation of Alcoholics Anonymous* (New York: Washington Square Press, 2005).

15. *"Pass It On."*

16. "Problem Drinkers," *March of Time*, 1946, http://www.aamuncie.org/March_of_Time_1946.html.

17. E. Kurtz, *Not-God: A History of Alcoholics Anonymous* (Center City, MN: Hazelden Educational Services, 1979), 92.

18. E. M. Jellinek, "Phases in the Drinking History of Alcoholics: Analysis of a Survey Conducted by the Official Organ of Alcoholics Anonymous," *Quarterly Journal of Studies on Alcohol* 7 (1946): 1–88.

19. T. J. Falcone, *Alcoholism: A Disease of Speculation* (Amsterdam, NY: Baldwin Research Institute, 2003), http://www.baldwinresearch.com/alcoholism.cfm.

20. Ad for *Alcoholics Anonymous*, http://www.barefootsworld.net/aa-medicine.html.

21. A. Tom Horvath, PhD, ABPP, "Court-Ordered 12-Step Attendance Is Illegal," *Practical Recovery*, http://practicalrecovery.com/readings/non-12-step-2/court-ordered.

22. *The Public Papers of the Presidents of the United States*, http://quod.lib.umich.edu/p/ppotpus/4731549.1966.001.

23. Federation of State Physician Health Programs website, http://www.fsphp.org/.

24. R. L. DuPont et al., "Setting the Standard for Recovery: Physicians' Health Programs," *Journal of Substance Abuse Treatment* 36 (2009): 159–71.

25. E. M. Gallas, "Endorsing Religion: Drug Courts and the 12-Step Recovery Support Program," *American University Law Review* 53, no. 5 (June 2004), http://digitalcommons.wcl.american.edu/cgi/viewcontent.cgi?article=1110&context=aulr.

CHAPTER THREE

1. Jason Koebler, "Diet Soda Linked to Depression in NIH Study," *US News & World Report*, http://www.usnews.com/.

2. G. Taubes, "Do We Really Know What Makes Us Healthy?" *New York Times Magazine*, September 16, 2007.

3. Ibid.

4. Ibid.

5. Deborah Dawson, PhD, "Recovery from Alcohol Dependence: Response to Commentaries," *Addiction* 100, no. 3 (March 2005): 296–98.

6. A. H. Thurstin et al., "The Efficacy of AA Attendance for Aftercare of Inpatient Alcoholics: Some Follow-up Data," *International Journal of the Addictions* 22 (1987): 1083–90.

7. *Alcoholics Anonymous*, 3rd ed. (New York: AA World Services, 1976), 58–60.

8. J. M. Brandsma et al., *Outpatient Treatment of Alcoholism: A Review and Comparative Study* (Baltimore: University Park Press, 1980).

9. C. D. Emrick, "Alcoholics Anonymous: Membership Characteristics and Effectiveness as Treatment," *Recent Developments in Alcoholism* 7 (1989): 37–53.

10. D. C. Walsh et al., "A Randomized Trial of Treatment Options for Alcohol-Abusing Workers," *New England Journal of Medicine* 325, no. 11 (September 12, 1991): 775–82. The paper explains:

> The average length of stay at the 10 hospitals (of which 2 accounted for 86 percent of the hospital assignments) was 23 days. . . . The participating hospitals described their programs in similar terms . . . held AA meetings at the hospital, and cited abstinence as the goal of treatment. . . . The third treatment option—referred to as "choice"—was one that involved the subjects in the planning of their treatment. . . . The subjects randomly assigned to a choice of treatments were not required to join AA or enter a hospital, although the staff of the employee-assistance program sometimes encouraged them to do one or the other, and were free to elect no treatment. . . . Of the 71 subjects in the choice group, 29 elected hospitalization in a total of five hospitals (average length of stay, 24.5 days), 33 went directly to AA, 3 chose outpatient psychotherapy (with a social worker, a psychiatrist, or a marriage counselor), and 6 opted for no organized help at all.

11. D. Sacket, *Canadian Medical Association Journal* 167, no. 4 (2002): 363–64, http://www.cmaj.ca/content/167/4/363.full.

12. *Cochrane Database Systems Review* 3 (July 2006): CD005032.

13. Citations from ibid.: Brown 2002; Cloud 2004; Davis 2002; Kahler 2004; MATCH 1998; McCrady 1996; Walsh 1991; Zemore 2004.

14. R. Fiorentine, "After Drug Treatment: Are 12-Step Programs Effective in Maintaining Abstinence?" *American Journal of Drug and Alcohol Abuse* 25, no. 1 (February 25, 1999): 93–116.

15. B. S. McCrady et al., "Issues in the Implementation of a Randomized Clinical Trial That Includes Alcoholics Anonymous: Studying AA-Related Behaviors During Treatment," *Journal of Studies on Alcohol and Drugs* 57 (1996): 604–12.

16. Quoted in Taubes, "Do We Really Know What Makes Us Healthy?"

17. Ibid.

18. R. H. Moos and B. S. Moos, "Paths of Entry into Alcoholics Anonymous: Consequences for Participation and Remission," *Alcoholism: Clinical and Experimental Research* 29, no. 10 (2005): 1858–68; R. H. Moos and B. S. Moos, "Participation in

Treatment and Alcoholics Anonymous: A 16-Year Follow-Up of Initially Un-treated Individuals," *Journal of Clinical Psychology* 62 (2006): 735–50.

19. Moos and Moos, "Participation in Treatment and Alcoholics Anonymous."

20. Ibid.

21. Ibid.

22. J. McKellar et al., "Predictors of Changes in Alcohol-Related Self-Efficacy over 16 Years," *Journal of Substance Abuse Treatment* 35, no. 2 (September 2008): 148–55.

23. C. Timko et al., "Driving While Intoxicated Among Individuals Initially Untreated for Alcohol Use Disorders: One- and Sixteen-Year Follow-ups," *Journal of Studies on Alcohol and Drugs* 72, no. 2 (March 2011): 173–84.

24. John-Kåre Vederhus and Øistein Kristensen, "High Effectiveness of Self-Help Programs after Drug Addiction Therapy," *BMC Psychiatry* 6, no. 35 (2006).

25. Jane Witbrodt et al., "Do 12-Step Meeting Attendance Trajectories over 9 Years Predict Abstinence?" *Journal of Substance Abuse Treatment* 43, no. 1 (July 2012): 30–43.

26. J. McKellar et al., "Alcoholics Anonymous Involvement and Positive Alcohol-Related Outcomes: Cause, Consequence, or Just a Correlate? A Prospective 2-Year Study of 2,319 Alcohol-Dependent Men," *Journal of Consulting and Clinical Psychology* 71, no. 2 (2003): 302–8.

27. E-mail to the author.

28. McKellar et al., "Alcoholics Anonymous Involvement."

29. L. Kaskutas et al., "Alcoholics Anonymous Effectiveness: Faith Meets Science," *Journal of Addictive Diseases* 28, no. 2 (2009): 145–57.

30. R. D. Weiss et al., "The Effect of 12-Step Self-Help Group Attendance and Participation on Drug Use Outcomes among Cocaine-Dependent Patients," *Drug and Alcohol Dependence* 77, no. 2 (2005):177–84.

31. John Majer et al., "12-Step Involvement among a U.S. National Sample of Oxford House Residents," *Journal of Substance Abuse Treatment* 41 (2011): 37–44.

32. M. Ferri et al., "Alcoholics Anonymous and Other 12-Step Programmes for Alcohol Dependence," *Cochrane Database Systems Review* 3 (July 2006): CD005032.

33. *Comments on A.A. Triennial Surveys* (New York: AA World Services, December 1990).

34. H. Fingarette, *Heavy Drinking: The Myth of Alcoholism as a Disease* (Berkeley: University of California Press, 1988).

35. J. Harris et al., "Prior Alcoholics Anonymous (AA) Affiliation and the Acceptability of the Twelve Steps to Patients Entering UK Statutory Addiction Treatment," *Journal of Studies on Alcohol* 64, no. 2 (2003): 257–61.

36. Fingarette, *Heavy Drinking*.

37. Fiorentine, "After Drug Treatment."

38. R. Shammas et al., "Remission in Rheumatoid Arthritis," *Current Rheumatology Reports* 12, no. 5 (October 2010): 355–62.

39. R. G. Smart, "Spontaneous Recovery in Alcoholics: A Review and Analysis of the Available Research," *Drug and Alcohol Dependence* 1 (1975–1976): 284.

40. Sheldon Zimberg, *The Clinical Management of Alcoholism* (New York: Brunner-Routledge, 1982).

41. S. E. Mueller et al., "The Impact of Self-Help Group Attendance on Relapse Rates after Alcohol Detoxification in a Controlled Study," *Alcohol and Alcoholism* 42, no. 2 (2007): 108–12.

42. G. E. Vaillant, *The Natural History of Alcoholism* (Cambridge, MA: Harvard University Press, 1983), 283.

43. R. B. Cutler and D. A. Fishbain, "Are Alcoholism Treatments Effective? The Project MATCH Data," *BMC Public Health* 14, no 5 (2005): 75.

44. D. Dawson et al., "Recovery from DSM-IV Alcohol Dependence: United States, 2001–2002," *Addiction* 100, no. 3 (2005): 281–92. *Dawson and colleagues' methodology is as follows:* "This analysis is based on data from the 2001–02 National Epidemiologic Survey on Alcohol and Related Conditions (NESARC), in which data were collected in personal interviews conducted with one randomly selected adult in each sample household. A subset of the NESARC sample (total n = 43 093), consisting of 4422 US adults 18 years of age and over classified with PPY DSM-IV alcohol dependence, were evaluated with respect to their past-year recovery status: past-year dependence, partial remission, full remission, asymptomatic risk drinking, abstinent recovery (AR) and non-abstinent recovery (NR)."

45. Brendan I. Koerner, "Secret of AA: After 75 Years, We Don't Know How It Works," *Wired*, June 23, 2010, http://www.wired.com/magazine/2010/06/ff_alcoholics_anonymous/.

CHAPTER FOUR

1. Hazelden website admissions page, http://www.hazelden.org/web/public/admissions.page.

2. Betty Ford Center website, http://www.bettyfordcenter.org.

3. Sierra Tucson website, http://www.sierratucson.com.

4. Flyer in author's collection.

5. Promises Treatment Centers website, http://www.promises.com.

6. Saint Jude Retreats website, http://www.soberforever.net.

7. Sheila Marikar, "Promises Kept, Promises Broken: Inside Hollywood's Preeminent Rehab Center," ABCNews.com, March 4, 2011, http://abcnews.go.com/entertainment/charlie-sheen-shines-light-promises-rehab-center-stars/story?id=13048850.

8. Lance Dodes, MD, "Why There Is Lunacy, Literally, In 28-Day Rehabs," *The Heart of Addiction* blog, *Psychology Today*, April 22, 2012, http://www.psychologytoday.com.

9. Paul Pringle, "The Trouble with Rehab, Malibu-Style," *Los Angeles Times*, October 9, 2007.

10. R. F. Forman and W. G. Bovasso, "Staff Beliefs about Addiction Treatment," *Journal of Substance Abuse Treatment* 21, no. 1 (July 2001): 1–9.

11. C. Russell et al., "Predictors of Addiction Treatment Providers' Beliefs in the Disease and Choice Models of Addiction," *Journal of Substance Abuse Treatment* 40, no. 2 (March 2011): 150–64.

12. Pringle, "The Trouble with Rehab."

13. Benedict Carey, "Drug Rehabilitation or Revolving Door?" *New York Times*, December 22, 2008.

14. "Outcomes of Alcohol/Other Drug Dependency Treatment," Butler Center for Research, February 2011, Hazelden website, http://www.hazelden.org/web/public/researchupdates.

15. R. Stitchfield and P. Owen, "Hazelden's Model of Treatment and Its Outcome," *Journal of Addictive Behaviors* 23, no. 5 (1998): 669–83.

16. Ibid.

17. Marikar, "Promises Kept, Promises Broken."

18. Dana-Farber Cancer Institute website, http://www.dana-farber.org; Austen Riggs Center website, http://www.austenriggs.org.

19. 1913 ad for Battle Creek Sanitarium, Google Images, www.google.com.

20. Ad for Dansville Sanitarium, Google Images, www.google.com.

21. Ad for Moore's Brook Sanitarium, Google Images, www.google.com.

CHAPTER FIVE

1. L. Robins et al., "Narcotic Use in Southeast Asia and Afterward," *Archives of General Psychiatry* 32 (1975): 955–61.

2. According to the US Centers for Disease Control and Prevention, the US adult population of smokers dropped by 40 percent between 1965 and 1990 ("Smoking Prevalence Among U.S. Adults, 1955–2010," *Infoplease*, 2012, http://www.infoplease.com/ipa/A0762370.html).

3. E. Khantzian, "The Self-Medication Hypothesis of Addictive Disorders: Focus on Heroin and Cocaine Dependence," *American Journal of Psychiatry* 142 (1985): 1259–64.

4. J. E. Grant et al., "Pathological Gambling and Alcohol Use Disorder," *Alcohol Research and Health* 26, no. 2 (2002): 143–50, pubs.niaaa.nih.gov/publications/arh26-2/143–150.pdfÐ.

5. E. Nestler, "From Neurobiology to Treatment: Progress against Addiction," *Nature Neuroscience* 5 (2002): 1076–79; http://www.ncbi.nlm.nih.gov/pubmed/12403990; P. Kalivas and N. Volkow, "The Neural Basis of Addiction: A Pathology of Motivation and Choice," *American Journal of Psychiatry* 152 (2005): 1303–13; N. Volkow et al., "Dopamine in Drug Abuse and Addiction," *Archives of Neurology* 64 (2007): 1475–79.

6. John E. Helzer, MD, "Significance of the Robins et al. Vietnam Veterans Study," *American Journal on Addictions* 19 (2010): 218–21.

7. Lance Dodes, MD, *The Heart of Addiction* (New York: HarperCollins, 2002).

8. K. Merikangas, "The Genetic Epidemiology of Alcoholism," *Psychological Medicine* 20 (1990): 11–22.

9. L. M. Dodes, "Compulsion and Addiction," *Journal of the American Psychoanalytic Association* 44 (1996): 815–35.

10. This is the mission of all psychotherapy: bringing factors to awareness and working them out to understand and eventually master the lingering issues in our emotional lives.

11. For those who would like to read more about these ideas and see many real-life examples of how they apply, please see *The Heart of Addiction* (n. 7) and my book *Breaking Addiction: A 7-Step Handbook to Ending Any Addiction* (New York: HarperCollins, 2011).

12. Indeed, the hiker Aron Ralston was widely hailed for cutting off his own arm to escape a boulder in 2003; the 2010 movie *127 Hours* chronicles and celebrates his bravery.

13. Dodes, *Breaking Addiction*.

CHAPTER SIX

1. Here's the full text of the post:

> I recently completed a review of the scientific literature about the effectiveness of 12-step programs, including regular AA meetings and AA-based rehab treatments. What I found is provocative: Although many people do well in 12-step programs and the famous rehabs around the country, most do not. I'm writing a wide-release book about these issues, to be published next year.
>
> What's missing from the project are the firsthand accounts of how people with addictions feel about their own experiences in 12-step recovery. That's where I hope to have help from readers of this blog: If you would like to describe your honest and open account of personal experiences in AA and/or rehab, I'd like to hear it. Please note that both positive and negative experiences are welcome. If you don't have a story to tell but know someone who might want to share, I would appreciate if you could pass this request along to them. If I receive enough accounts, I intend to publish many of them verbatim in the forthcoming book.
>
> No identifying information will be published, including any information about individual counselors, treaters or sponsors. (I.e., it's fine to say "I was treated at Betty Ford Treatment Center" but not "I was treated by John Smith, a counselor at Betty Ford.")
>
> If you'd like to participate in this project, please contact me directly at 12stepbook@gmail.com. Let me know in the email how you'd like to be contacted, and whether you would prefer to conduct a phone interview or simply send your written thoughts. Thank you, and I look forward to hearing from you.

CHAPTER SEVEN

1. R. Bond et al., "A 61-Million-Person Experiment in Social Influence and Political Mobilization," *Nature* 489 (2012): 295–98.

2. L. Kaskutas, "Alcoholics Anonymous Effectiveness: Faith Meets Science," *Journal of Addictive Diseases* 28, no. 2 (2009): 145–57.

3. R. H. Moos and B. S. Moos, "Participation in Treatment and Alcoholics Anonymous: A 16-Year Follow-Up of Initially Untreated Individuals," *Journal of Clinical Psychology* 62 (2006): 735–50.

4. Kevin Gray, "Does AA Really Work? A Round-Up of Recent Studies," *The Fix*, January 29, 2012, http://www.thefix.com/.

5. J. Harris et al., "Prior Alcoholics Anonymous (AA) Affiliation and the Acceptability of the Twelve Steps to Patients Entering UK Statutory Addiction Treatment," *Journal of Studies on Alcohol* 64, no. 2 (2003): 257–61.

6. Ibid.

7. Poster from the Center on Alcoholism, Substance Abuse, and Addictions, J. Scott Tonigan, Clinical Research Branch, Center on Alcoholism, Substance Abuse, and Addictions (CASAA), University of New Mexico.

8. P. L. Owen et al., "Participation in Alcoholics Anonymous: Intended and Unintended Change Mechanisms," *Alcohol: Clinical and Experimental Research* 27, no. 3 (March 2003): 524–32.

9. National Clergy Conference on Alcoholism, *The "Blue Book"* 12 (1960): 179–210, http://www.silkworth.net/religion_clergy/01052.html.

10. J. Markham, "Does Mandatory AA/NA Violate the First Amendment?" *North Carolina Criminal Law* (blog), October 16, 2009, http://nccriminallaw.sog.unc.edu/?p=784.

11. Griffin v. Coughlin, 88 N.Y. 2d 674 (1996), 673 N.E.2d 98, 649 N.Y.S.2d 903, June 11, 1996.

12. J. Kelly et al., "Negative Affect, Relapse, and Alcoholics Anonymous (AA): Does AA Work by Reducing Anger?" *Journal of Studies on Alcohol and Drugs* 71 (2010): 434–44.

13. J. Tonigan and S. Rice, "Is It Beneficial to Have an Alcoholics Anonymous Sponsor?" *Psychology of Addictive Behaviors* 24 (2010): 397–403.

14. P. C. Bernhardt et al., "Testosterone Changes during Vicarious Experiences of Winning and Losing Among Fans at Sporting Events," *Physiology and Behavior* 65, no. 1 (August 1998): 59–62.

CHAPTER EIGHT

1. *Twelve Steps and Twelve Traditions* (New York: AA World Services, 1952), 42.

2. For many examples of this, see my book *Breaking Addiction: A 7-Step Handbook for Ending Any Addiction* (New York: HarperCollins, 2011).

3. Clarence Snyder, *Going Through the Steps*, AA sponsorship pamphlet, 1944.

CHAPTER NINE

1. C. Timko and A. DeBenedetti, "A Randomized Controlled Trial of Intensive Referral to 12-Step Self-Help Groups: One-Year Outcomes," *Drug and Alcohol Dependence* 90 (2007): 270–79.

2. Li-Tzy Wu et al., "How Do Prescription Opioid Users Differ From Users of Heroin or Other Drugs in Psychopathology?" *Journal of Addiction Medicine* 5, no. 1 (March 2011): 28–35.

3. Sarah W. Yip et al., "Health/Functioning Characteristics, Gambling Behaviors, and Gambling-Related Motivations in Adolescents Stratified by Gambling Problem Severity: Findings from a High School Survey," *American Journal on Addictions* 20, no. 6 (November–December 2011): 495–508.

4. Betty Ford Institute Consensus Panel, "What Is Recovery? A Working Definition from the Betty Ford Institute," *Journal of Substance Abuse Treatment* 33, no. 3 (October 2007): 221–28.

5. C. Rutger et al., "Effect of Alcohol References in Music on Alcohol Consumption in Public Drinking Places," *American Journal on Addictions* 20, no. 6 (November–December 2011): 530–34.

6. Igor Elman et al., "Psychosocial Stress and Its Relationship to Gambling Urges in Individuals with Pathological Gambling," *American Journal on Addictions* 19, no. 4 (July–August 2010): 332–39.

7. R. B. Cutler and D. A. Fishbain, "Are Alcoholism Treatments Effective? The Project MATCH Data," *BMC Public Health* 14, no. 5 (2005): 75.

8. Lance Dodes, MD, *Breaking Addiction: A 7-Step Handbook for Ending Any Addiction* (New York: HarperCollins, 2011).

9. J. P. A. Ioannidis, "Why Most Published Research Findings Are False," *PLOS Medicine* 2, no. 8 (2005), http://www.plosmedicine.org/article/info:doi/10.1371/journal.pmed.0020124.

10. Nate Silver, *The Signal and the Noise: Why So Many Predictions Fail—But Some Don't* (New York: Penguin Press, 2012).

11. Ioannidis, "Why Most Published Research Findings Are False."

12. Ibid.

13. P. W. Anderson, "More Is Different: Broken Symmetry and the Nature of the Hierarchical Structure of Sciences," *Science* 177, no. 4047 (1972): 393–96.

14. Dodes, *Breaking Addiction*.

INDEX

abstinence: correlation with engagement, 51; counting days of, 136–137; percentage of days abstinent (PDA), 74–75; relationship with TSF, 47; reported rates of, 72; sponsorship unrelated to, 126

addiction, 81–95; biological views of, 85–88, 147–148, 152, 155–156; compulsion model of, 83–85, 89–90; consequences of, 134–135; as failure of morality, 5–6, 13, 98–99, 110; as form of insanity, 144–145; geneticists' views of, 88–89, 147, 155–156; higher brain functions and, 87–88; as innate, 139; myths about (*See* addiction myths); physical v. psychological, 81, 82–85; psychological precipitants of, 156–157; psychology of (*See* psychology of addiction); soldiers in Vietnam War, 83–84, 86–87; studies of treatments (*See* addiction treatment studies); as substitute for helplessness, 91–92, 127; understanding, 81–82, 156–157

addiction counselors, 69–70, 142–144

addiction myths, 134–146; character defects of addicts, 141–142, 145; counting days of abstinence, 136–137; denial myth, 144–145; "hitting bottom," 134–135; insanity myth, 144; 90/90 prescription, 140–141; "one day at a time," 139; "one-size-fits-all" treatment, 137–138; peer group influence,

139–140; surrendering, 135–136; value of addicts as counselors, 142–144

addiction switches, 85, 93, 108

addiction treatment studies, 29–57. *See also specific studies*; claims of 12-step programs and, 34–36; Cochrane Collaboration review, 36–40; compliance effect, 32–33, 39, 40, 41–42; controlled (randomized) (*See* controlled studies); definition of success, 33–34; demographics of, 49; designing perfect study, 150–151, 158–160; determining actual success rates, 1–2, 52–53, 73–74; dropout rates and, 44–50; evidence-based studies as mirage, 151–157; failure of, 147–160; failure to study psychology of addiction, 152–153; human studies, special considerations in, 29–31; of identical twins, 89; ineffectiveness of AA, 56–57; lack of, 147–151; longitudinal, 41, 42, 43–44, 151; observational (*See* observational studies); problem of spontaneous remission, 53–55; project MATCH, 55–56, 150; publication of, limited in scope, 148, 157–158; question of spirituality, 124–125; role of motivation, 50–52; statistics ineffectual in, 157–158

addicts: as addiction counselors, 69–70, 142–144; character defects of, 141–142, 145; demeaning treatment of, 99–100, 137–138, 143–144; need for individual evaluation of, 132–133